EBURY PRESS
PAUSE, REWIND

Nawaz Modi Singhania trained, taught and was certified in the US as a fitness professional by the American Council on Exercise (ACE) and International Dance Exercise Association (IDEA) in the early 1990s.

Upon her return to India, she founded a fitness centre under the brand name Body Art, which provides its members with holistic mind, body, spiritual, emotional and psychological fitness programmes.

Nawaz has participated in fitness conferences, workshops and conventions in the US, Australia, the UK, Singapore and Hong Kong. She is a columnist and has written for various online and offline publications, including *Mid-Day*, *Femina*, *Times of India*, *Bombay Times*, *Mumbai Mirror*, *Hello*, *India Today*, *Hindustan Times*, *DNA*, *Deccan Chronicle*, *Cosmopolitan*, *Health & Fitness*, *Business World*, *G2* and others. She is interviewed regularly on various radio channels on fitness, health and lifestyle-related matters. She has appeared on various fitness shows as a judge and trainer, and on India's biggest fitness channel on Tata Sky—Active Fitness—as a fitness expert and show host.

Pause, Rewind is her first book.

Celebrating 35 Years of
Penguin Random House India

PAUSE, REWIND

Natural
Anti-Ageing
Techniques

Nawaz Modi Singhania

EBURY
PRESS

An imprint of Penguin Random House

EBURY PRESS

USA | Canada | UK | Ireland | Australia
New Zealand | India | South Africa | China | Singapore

Ebury Press is part of the Penguin Random House group of companies
whose addresses can be found at global.penguinrandomhouse.com

Published by Penguin Random House India Pvt. Ltd
4th Floor, Capital Tower 1, MG Road,
Gurugram 122 002, Haryana, India

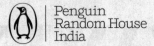

Penguin
Random House
India

First published in Ebury Press by Penguin Random House India 2023

Copyright © Nawaz Modi Singhania 2023

ISBN 9780143460602

Neither the author nor the publishers of *Pause, Rewind* are doctors or medical care
providers and have no expertise in diagnosing, examining, or treating medical conditions
of any kind, or in determining the effect of any specific exercise on a medical condition.
The information and exercises provided in this book are for reference only and are to be
used under professional guidance. They are not offered as a replacement or substitute for
professional medical advice or treatment or the direct guidance of a qualified instructor.
Not all exercises are suitable for everyone, and making use of this or any other exercise
programme may result in injury. Always, in your particular case, consult a doctor
and obtain full medical clearance before practising any exercise programme. Exercise
programmes must always be practised under the direct supervision of a qualified
instructor. Practising under the direct supervision and guidance of a qualified instructor
may reduce the risk of injury. Not all exercise programmes are suitable for all people.
Practising under the direct supervision and guidance of a qualified instructor, in addition
to the direction of your doctor, can also help determine what poses are suitable for your
particular case. The author, publishers and distributors assume no responsibility or
liability for any injuries or losses that may result from any exercise programme, or from
the adoption of any instruction or advice expressed in this book. The author, publishers
and distributors make no representations or warranties with regards to the completeness
or accuracy of the information contained in this book.

Typeset in Sabon by Manipal Technologies Limited, Manipal
Printed at Thomson Press India Ltd, New Delhi

www.penguin.co.in

MIX
Paper from
responsible sources
FSC® C010615

Contents

Foreword

My wellness guide, Nawaz Modi Singhania, is an important name in the fitness sector. She has been working in this field for the last several years and is passionate about promoting health and wellness among the youth. Many years before the culture of fitness centres had become a part of urban lifestyle, as a step forward in this direction, Nawaz started fitness centres in Mumbai under the brand name of Body Art Fitness Centre. With the help of print and electronic media, she has put in painstaking efforts to make people aware about holistic fitness, healthy lifestyles and wellness. During the Covid-19 lockdown, she helped people stay healthy via live group Zoom classes and online personal training. With her heavyweight years of experience in this field, she has penned this book titled *Time Arrest: Natural Anti-Ageing Techniques,* which is very appropriate and talks about all aspects of anti-ageing, health and well-being. I trust that this book will guide readers of all ages and create awareness about the right nutritional practices, types and ways to exercise.

In the Indian culture, a balanced and adequate diet has always been considered to be of paramount importance in order to attain healthful, spiritual living. According to Vedic beliefs, the human body is a divine gift and it is our duty to protect and secure our body by practising healthy living and appropriate eating practices. Accordingly, the food we eat has been given the divine place as *Purnabramha*.

Change is the only thing that is permanent in nature. Changing lifestyles have brought about a sea of change in food options in India, over and above the traditional ones. These new options have dragged in with them new challenges with respect to nutrition and health issues for the Indian population. Apart from the introduction of new food options, a shift in lifestyle has also brought with it varying eating patterns, with an increase in snacking, skipping meals, not eating meals in a family setting, eating out and ordering in. These unhealthy lifestyles and eating patterns of choosing fast food over healthy and traditional foods are now showing up in the form of obesity, morbidities, mental health issues, early ageing, etc.

Today, India is going through a phase of economic transition, and while malnutrition and undernutrition continue to be a major problem, the prevalence of over-nutrition is also emerging as a significant issue, especially in urban areas. For the Indian youth, it is high time they tune into healthy lifestyles and eating habits. Against this backdrop, personalities like Nawaz Modi Singhania, who have been engaged in the fitness sector for a long time, can guide people of all ages and introduce them to a wellness mantra.

I wish Nawaz every success with this book and also for her future projects.

—**Amruta Devendra Fadnavis**
3 June 2023

Introduction

First off, I'd like to set the tone for this book by narrating a story. Anyone who knows my husband Gautam or knows of him, is aware of his passion for cars and racing. When he was in his teens, he was out one day in London, looking to buy a safety racing helmet. He walked into a store that sold racing gear. While looking around at the wide array of helmets on display, he got thoroughly confused. The pricing ranged hugely, from really low-cost ones to insanely expensive helmets, with their prices in the stratosphere. It was difficult for him to decipher which was the right one for him to buy. Every helmet's job would be to protect the head anyway, right? So why such a large spectrum to select from? The salesman saw the confusion on Gautam's face, walked up to him and asked if he could be of any help. Gautam stated that he was not sure which helmet to buy due to the wide cost variant and asked what the right amount would be to spend. The salesman smiled and simply replied, 'Sir, that depends on the value you place on your own head!'

That one sharp school-of-hard-knocks reply that the salesman gave to Gautam holds the key to several answers in our life. No matter what you do for a living, the value you place on yourself, on your own head, will always determine the quality of the life you live. And I say 'quality', not 'quantity', because living longer does not necessarily mean living better.

Having said that, all of us want to be young forever and a day. That's why it is important not to wait till the first wrinkle or the first sign of hair thinning, to start halting the process of ageing. Instead, aim for a healthy, youthful, active life—such that running a marathon at sixty-five or doing yoga in your eighties isn't intimidating or a laughable dream. That is what this book is all about—living an active life that isn't limited to performing physical endeavours but also makes you enjoy your days to the fullest.

As someone who has been in the fitness industry for decades, founding Body Art—India's premier, leading fitness centres—way before fitness became a fad and seeing this luxury become a necessity, I felt compelled to write a book that would guide you to live that life. It is written with the intention of tapping into your inner self to get you moving every single day and to truly enjoy balanced, wholesome, nutritious and delicious meals without thinking of this as a 'diet you *must* follow', keeping you captured and tortured in a 'diet jail'! It is written for you to take care of your skin, body, mind, soul and psyche—essentially through exercise and nutrition—because you truly love yourself so much. It is about living your best life and becoming your best self—youthful, full of energy, vibrant and being in the best possible health.

It is written for you to develop a positive outlook towards life, radiating such confidence that no matter what stage of life you are in or how cloudy the days are, once you've read this book, you will aim to be your own sunshine. Through this book, you will learn the methods of managing stress and time better—often through simple breath control and exercises that make for a healthier lifestyle. It is written for you to be perfect, impressive and unforgettable at any age, even when the signs and symptoms lean towards the golden years. It is written to empower you to live a life of gratitude, resilience, with a positive attitude, courage and enlightenment, overcoming stereotypes and being a model of optimal living.

Above all, it is written to motivate you to look and be your best self, while living your best life at any age.

Welcome aboard this journey of arresting time and being forever young!

1

Exercise and Its Significance

Get moving . . . now

Everyone in my family has very bad eyesight. My father, at the tender age of five, wore thick glasses with a power of five for his myopia. He told me that it was heartbreaking for his family to see him with such a thick pair of glasses on the bridge of such a young child's nose. I, on the other hand, had 20/20 vision when I was a kid. Usually, people get reading glasses by the time they turn forty. So the moment I turned forty, I made an appointment to get my eyes tested by the highly acclaimed ophthalmologist, Dr Burjor Banaji, at his clinic in Fort, Mumbai. First, his nurse took down my medical history, asking questions like— do you find yourself squinting when reading? Do you find it difficult to read menus in dimly-lit restaurants? Do you move your reading material back and forth somewhat to be able to focus and read easily? Do you get headaches? The answers to all these questions were 'No'.

Perplexed, she asked me, 'Then why have you come?'

I said, 'Because I just turned forty and considering most people get reading glasses by that time, I thought it best I get checked.'

She nodded in agreement as she then ushered me into the doctor's cabin. When he read my age on the notes the nurse had just taken, he said I'd definitely need glasses. But when he finished testing, he said, 'Nawaz, you are not even within sniffing distance of glasses!'

I asked curiously, 'But you just said that since I have now turned forty, I would definitely need them.'

He replied, 'That's true. But you see, you are very fit and healthy, therefore all your organs and system are ageing very slowly. You're very well preserved.'

Pondering over that, I said, 'I don't really do any eye exercises. I do facial exercises and for the body of course, but have never done any specific eye exercises per se or for the optic nerves or associated muscles in particular.'

He replied, 'That doesn't matter, even if you don't work out something in particular, because of your overall wellness and fitness, everything ages much more slowly.'

The good doctor asked me to see him again in a couple of years, saying by then I probably would need glasses, so once again, I religiously did just that. I had a déjà vu moment with the nurse because yet again she ran me through her whole checklist of predictable questions and once again I had zero complaints. Again, she wondered why I was even there. When I was bustled into the doctor's cabin, he smiled and matter-of-factly said, 'Yes, by now you should need glasses.'

However, when he checked my eyesight, he said, 'Nawaz, your eyes are in showroom condition. If you keep this up a bit longer, there's a good chance you'll never need glasses—reading or otherwise.'

This was a big eye-opener to me, because what is more important in terms of the benefits of exercise than having optimal eyesight? Our eyes are the windows through which we view our whole world. Known to be the windows to our soul, the eyes are the most important of all our senses. But we take eyesight for granted. We are always so focused on the fat loss, inch loss, weight loss, toning up, stamina and so many other benefits of exercise, that we are blind to this fact. Pun intended, of course!

Benefits of Regular Exercise

There is a plethora of benefits of consistent exercise. Regardless of age, gender and physical ability, everyone gains from exercise. Besides fat and inch loss, which most people associate with exercising, you get increased strength, endurance, stamina, flexibility and muscle tone. With exercise, you can move more easily and quickly, and perform several tasks comfortably, without getting fatigued or injured. You attain the right physical proportion and body composition as well. When you exercise, your body releases the 'feel good' or the 'happy hormones', such as endorphin, serotonin and dopamine, that trigger a positive feeling in the body, similar to that of morphine. They are powerful anti-depressant hormones, often even more effective than antidepressant medications.[1] Endorphins interact with the receptors in your brain to reduce your perception of pain, leaving you feeling happier, more relaxed and less anxious. Your sleep improves immensely, your mental alertness and self-confidence are at an all-time high, and you radiate a healthy halo, wherein you don't get or look fatigued through the day.

In addition, being active boosts high-density lipoprotein (HDL) cholesterol (good cholesterol) and decreases unhealthy triglycerides, thus decreasing your risk of cardiovascular diseases. Problems including stroke, high blood pressure, type 2 diabetes, depression, anxiety, many types of cancer, arthritis and falls are kept under check. Mayo Clinic states that, 'Regular, daily physical activity can lower the risk of heart disease. Physical activity helps control your weight. It also reduces the chances of developing other conditions that may put a strain on the heart, such as high blood pressure, high cholesterol and type 2 diabetes.'[2]

Then again, exercise is best known to reverse common signs of ageing, including an unsteady gait, balance-related issues, knee problems, back problems, postural deviations, urinary incontinence, bowel control and eyesight. It gives the immune system a major boost. After all, the pandemic has taught us that keeping physically and mentally healthy, keeping our cardio-respiratory system in prime condition, and increasing our immunity, just must be each individual's top priority at all times—so what's not to love about exercise?

The Right Route

Different forms of exercise are a mix of high- and low-impact routines, and these include cardio dance classes, step aerobics, box-aerobics, Zumba, sculpting, toning and strength-training using dumbbells, weighted bars and plates, new body formats, using light weights, mat Pilates, calisthenics, Callanetics, trampoline workouts, indoor biking, muscle ballet, slide training, Swiss ball, facial fitness/anti-ageing, aqua aerobics, aqua yoga, spinning, circuit training, functional fitness, chair workouts, yoga, yogalates, gyrokinesis and so much more. You must cross-train or take up different workouts regularly to ensure continuous progress so that you don't stagnate.

My advice to you would be to consult a fitness professional to get a bespoke plan, tailor-made to your requirements. Health applications which do the same at very affordable rates are a great alternative. This is important as, when you start a programme, your fitness levels, health limitations (if any), goals, age, previous experience with exercise, even likes and dislikes, etc., must be taken into consideration. One size never fits all. A trainer can teach you the right technique, correct your alignment and figure out the appropriate intensity level for you since it varies for each person.

Also, remember to check with your medical practitioner before starting a new exercise programme, especially if you have any concerns about your fitness levels, if you haven't exercised for a long time, or you have acute or chronic health problems, such as heart disease, diabetes or arthritis.

Get Started . . .

Need more convincing to get moving? It doesn't matter whether you have a large chunk of time in the day to exercise or not. Remember that any amount of activity is better than none at all. Consistency is key. Not everyone needs to prepare to run a marathon, but everyone would certainly benefit from walking every day. It's okay to start small. Tell yourself that. You don't always need weights and heavy equipment— sometimes makeshift items that you can find in your home like a band, *dupatta*, book, ball, chair or towel are enough. Remove all your mental blocks. Take baby steps: park your car further from your destination, avoid elevators, walk to stores in a nearby radius and track your steps to make it all collectively effective for you. And now that you have this book, you know that can start from the comfort of your bedroom.

2

Motivation for Ageing Well

Because happiness is a choice

Human souls are filled with aspirations. Our lists of needs and desires never seem to end, and we seem to be in a constant rush to keep chasing them. In this process, health—the actual premise of our existence—is the most ignored. The motivation to become healthier and fitter is all around us. For some, it is the physical and mental pain of being overweight. For others, it is the realization that time is marching forward and/or that they have young ones and hence must be prudent enough to take good care of their own health. Sometimes it is about weight-related fertility issues, Polycystic Ovarian Disease (PCOD) or a chronic medical condition like diabetes or arthritis. In many cases, it is just about wanting to look good or feeling the pressure because of being in the public eye. I think whatever it is that motivates you to lead a healthy lifestyle, you must find your pressing reason and work towards it.

My Personal Back Story

For me, this realization came in many forms. I started out as a tiny little girl who was small-framed, fragile, weak and unable to do things that required too much physical labour. Over various incidents, there was always that realization that I wouldn't survive to adulthood if I continued in that fashion. I needed to get fitter and healthier before it was too late. Everyone has experiences that change their lives forever—for me, it was when I had my first child. I had put on weight quite easily and didn't like it at all. I started looking older and felt horrible—postnatal depression had a lot to do with all of this. It felt awful and I wanted my old self back. It didn't help that I was in the fitness industry, where I was looked up to as a mentor, and I didn't want to let go of that.

In the long run, what helped the most were the small changes. For instance, by rearranging my schedule, I managed somehow to get a short workout every day, even if it was with my baby in the crib right next to me. Or by tackling postnatal hair-fall by the horns and taking a trichologist's advice and treatment. Or managing to get adequate sleep by getting family or other help to fill in, to allow for a restful night. Over time, I did get back to a fitter state than pre-pregnancy.

Moving ahead, I had the same experience again with my second pregnancy. It was much harder because I was older, but I wanted the child just as much. Hence, I was happy to put in more effort on my part and felt much more motivated. Even after achieving my target, I never stopped working at being fit in this intensive way because it had worked well for me. It continues to make me feel so much better and so I keep at it.

The famous Henry Ford quote, 'Whether you think you can, or think you can't, you're right!'[3] really says it all. Winning or losing all happens only in the mind. The subsequent playing out of a situation can most often be traced back to your own intrinsic belief about yourself.

Good Thoughts, Good Words, Good Deeds

From the beginning, we as Zoroastrians are taught the virtues of good thoughts, good words and good deeds. It is hardwired into our psyche. The real power of choice or the true ability to make every decision day after day, be it small or mammoth, when standing at the crossroads of your life, lies at the level of thoughts. Thoughts become things—whatever you have in your life is because you first thought of it. Whether it is who you want to be, which friends you want to make, how many children you want to have, which college you want to study in, where you want to live, what kind of job you want to bag, which car you want to drive, who you want to marry, what your life goals are or where you want to holiday—every single thing is at first just a thought. The thought becomes the word, the word becomes the deed and then it materializes into whatever it is that you wanted. So that free will—that first seed—is only at the level of thought. After that, it is merely a chain reaction. Oftentimes, we are not very careful and mindful of our thoughts. We need to guard them sacredly and gatekeep our thoughts—what we allow in our mind and what we don't. Problems arise when there is no screening—when we are not mindful of what we see, read or hear. All those things become thoughts and that leads to positivity or negativity around us. These can manifest in a variety of ways—physical, emotional, mental, psychological. They tend to show up in our relationships and environment, becoming all-pervasive and having a spillover effect into every facet of life.

Invest in Yourself

It is easier to stay positive when we invest in ourselves. Nobody was born perfect and we are all works in progress. We all need to devote time and effort to plough into ourselves in different ways. As we get better with whatever we put ourselves into, we automatically begin to feel better about ourselves. Suddenly, we are not that negative anymore. Depression or that sinking feeling of sadness is no longer our normal. Exercise and movement help us stay positive. All those happy hormones get a huge boost with exercise, playing an ample role in keeping the spirits high and you happy.

Always Give Back

Another very important aspect that I've found in my own experience and also something I've learnt from my father, is the importance of giving back. Back in the day when I finished college, I was wondering what next to do with my life—if I should go the family way and be a lawyer or whether I should take up something else. I had multiple interests. My father told me that I'd never have the need to earn money, so I did not need to stress about that. Instead, he encouraged me to focus on doing something that would make me useful in society and allowed me to give back to people in a way that they couldn't easily get otherwise, in my own unique way. He spurred me on to put my life into giving back and a very large part of what I do is focused precisely on this. When you do things for others, you don't feel negative, regardless of whatever else might have been happening in your life. It is very self-healing, which also ties in with why I do what I do. I read somewhere that you always end up teaching that which you need to learn the most and that's what happened to me with regard to fitness and wellness.

Make a Gratitude List

Keeping a gratitude list is very important and effective. The more you jot down, the more you'll notice good things coming your way—it's just the law of the universe—like attracts like. By doing this, you change the energy in your headspace and in your heart. I am forever grateful for all of it—for whom and for what I have in my life.

Early Life

I was born underweight with the umbilical cord wrapped around my neck several times over. I was white as a sheet and wasn't breathing—they thought I was stillborn. Somehow, against all odds, I survived. I was small, weak and had a mitral valve prolapse (a genetic cardiac condition which affects the mitral valve between the left heart chambers, leading to an improper closure of the valve between the upper and lower heart chambers). I have worked slowly towards getting stronger, fitter and more able.

When I was ten years old, my parents split up. I remained with my father and my brothers. It was an awful time. I was a pre-teen, my body was undergoing various changes and I didn't know what to do. It was very awkward and there was no woman in the house to guide me on all things female. My grandparents lived in the flat next door, but my grandmother was dying of cancer, and so was in no condition to be of any help to me in these matters.

I started emotional binge eating—a subconscious way of coping. I realized much later in life that my emotions were deeply connected with my eating disorder. It had knocked my self-esteem down a peg or two and made me gain weight, lose my health, look older than my (then young) years and feel far worse. It dawned on me that eating to somehow feel better was actually hurting me much more than it was helping! The self-realization was very important in being able to stack up on whether this was serving me or sinking me. It enabled me to make wiser choices for my own best interest.

I was close to my mother and was supposed to leave with her after the divorce, but an incident occurred that made me change my mind about that. I felt that, as a young kid, I actually stood up to the situation and showed a lot of strength of character by being there for my two brothers and my father as they were falling apart in different ways, as I was too. I would be the one telling them that things were going to be okay. They, in their own ways, were struggling to make the best of a bad situation and were trying very hard to be there for me too.

Slowly, I started seeing the good in things. I realized that once my mother was gone, I got to rule the roost by running the house, the kitchen, managing the staff and calling the shots, all by default. My proverbial dark clouds had very large silver linings.

When I am low, I think back on the time that I was born and of how touch-and-go and bleak that time was. I remember that however bad things can sometimes be now, they are a zillion times better than back then. I think it sometimes helps to start from right down there at the bottom of the well, because from there, the only place to look at, is up—things can only get better. The thought is beautifully worded somewhere—why would a person choose to sit at the bottom of a well, when God has given them two strong arms to pull themselves up and out?

Good and bad happens to all of us. It is a part and parcel of living on planet Earth. One has to learn to deal with the downside of things in a much healthier fashion, process and metabolize them (if you will) in time, and come out stronger, wiser and healthier. That's the goal.

The Value of Hobbies

There is deep value in having leisure-related pursuits. Up until now, they were more of a casual pastime for me. I didn't realize up until lockdown what these pastimes actually were all about, in terms of depth and grounding. Being in the house full-time, I took up painting, composing and playing music. I was also consuming great educational content, doing an online business course with Harvard Business School, writing this book and I found myself more actively engaged with my kids and more. It all helped me connect with myself.

Happiness is a Choice

I don't let the things that I can't do get in the way of things that I can do. When I look at who and what I am, I feel humbled and deeply grateful for my blessings, especially when I see all that is happening around us in this fast-changing world.

I try to surround myself with people who are better and more accomplished than me, because I can learn from them and they inspire me. Surround yourself with people who will take you to different levels as opposed to those who are just yes-men or those who emotionally drain you. I feel so pleased when my friends do well—I don't feel any negativity. In fact, I turn around and proudly comment on what they've done and on how great I feel about the concerned persons. They motivate me to push myself above and beyond. This makes a world of a difference. Happiness is an internal job—it flows from inside out, not outside in. Nobody but you alone can make yourself happy. So go ahead and do the things that make you happier! Fill up your emotional, psychological and mental well with all things good!

3

Fitness and Self-Esteem

Building a better body image, for life

Fitness is all about mental, emotional, psychological and physical well-being—you cannot separate one from another. The approach to health must therefore necessarily be holistic in nature.

Fitness and self-esteem are bedfellows, depending on and feeding off each other. The rule is simple. The fitter you are, the more self-esteem and confidence you'll have. Also, the more self-esteem and confidence you have, the fitter you would *want* to be. One doesn't exist without the other. Fundamentally, it is your view of yourself and hence your relationship with yourself, that dictates how you relate to the world, the people and the things in it. In a more glamour-based world, to a great degree, how people treat and view you, the respect you command (or not) in all arenas of life—including the family space, friend circles, work colleagues, the community at large, etc.—depends upon your physical appearance or more importantly, on how you *feel* about yourself. Even the things that we think and say are hugely affected by this. The science of it is that besides helping you slip into your old dress or pair of jeans, exercise can boost your self-esteem and put you in a healthier and happier state of mind. And that's what you should be aiming for.

The Stress Buster

Exercise releases the feel-good or the happy hormones—specifically endorphins, serotonin and dopamine. Research shows that regular aerobic or cardio exercise decreases levels of stress, tension and depression. It elevates and stabilizes the mood, improves self-esteem and enhances sleep quality. These are only a few amongst the many improvements related to betterment of health, invariably reducing the levels of stress of an individual. Over time, you'll see that as little as five minutes of cardio or aerobic exercise will begin to stimulate the anti-anxiety effects in your body. In fact, with exercise, there's more to it than meets the eye. Things that you may think are unrelated to fitness are actually interconnected. For instance, with regular exercise, our blood pressure stays low, blood sugar is in control, heart disease remains at bay, and the less you weigh, the less the chance of suffering from diabetes, arthritis, etc. It's a virtual circle—when your overall health improves, you feel less stress.

Grey Matter Booster

Exercise has a great impact—not just on the body but also on the mind. Besides increasing muscle strength, cardio and muscle endurance, exercise gives you the energy to be clearer in your thoughts, to think afresh and to come up with new ideas. The hormones that are released during exercise (endorphins mostly) are in charge of improving the prioritizing functions of the brain. So, with exercise, you end up blocking out distractions—you think better, sharper and clearer, and are able to focus on the task at hand. It also sharpens your memory. The more you move around, the more energized you feel in the body and the mind. Even about fifteen minutes of generally moving around—even if it is walking about in your living room or doing knee lifts, marching or on-the-spot kicks—will give you a lot more energy on a cellular level. And guess what? That's what the mind is made up of. Cells.

Post exercise, you'll find that you're able to concentrate with a much clearer focus. The cerebral matter is able to improve upon itself and that is due to additional blood flow (circulation), through which proteins, minerals, vitamins and oxygen are delivered to the brain. When you work on a project post-workout, you have so much energy. You are sharper, more focused and your thoughts are clearer as they're coming from a place you didn't know existed. Importantly, the brain ages much more slowly when you are physically active. This means that you'll be steering off dementia,

Alzheimer's and other mental degenerative disorders just by being physically mobile and active.

Begin. Now.

Often, the biggest hurdle related to fitness is where to begin. The only answer to it is—start where you stand. It doesn't matter how unfit you may be today, make sure that every day is better than the last. Take steps in the right direction to ensure that, even if it's a little bit at a time, you improve your fitness in various ways. Whether it's cardio-respiratory or muscle fitness, working on your flexibility, posture and gait, balance or control, or getting that stubborn fat, inches and weight off—there are many aspects to fitness. You just need to know what your body needs and work towards getting fitter in that direction. The rest will follow.

Partner With None

I don't recommend exercising with a friend ever, for the same reason I don't recommend a partner at work. They come in because they think they have certain weaknesses and that leads them to consciously or otherwise lean on their partners or use them as crutches. When each one comes in with that notion, you can see what a recipe for disaster that's going to make! This never works. People tend to rely more on each other rather than take up their load themselves. That's a recipe for disappointment and failure right there.

If your friend doesn't show up one day, if he/she is unwell, has something else to do or simply isn't feeling up to it, you're likely to drop out of the workout session yourself. That's not okay. You should be self-reliant. The will to stay fit lasts longer this way versus when you are dependent on a friend. A personal trainer, on the other hand, is a good idea because he/she will regulate your regimen and you'll be more committed. For instance, you know that 10 to 11 a.m. on Monday, Wednesday and Friday is your slot with your trainer, and there is nothing you can do to get out of it. You've paid good money for it, you'll prioritize it and ensure that you journal it. Tick that box and show up!

Being Regular

Journal your fitness regime and make it a habit. Just like you sleep every night, brush your teeth regularly and have a bath every day, exercising is something that you've *got* to do. You have to realize that exercising is as important as breathing or eating—prioritize it the same way. However, let it become a part of your day and your system without you having to think too much about it. While it is true that we get run over by too many pressures and can't always put in the same sort of time or energy to exercise, short, compressed 2–3 minute compound workouts are a good enough substitute, rather than nothing at all. For instance, do two or three sets of planks to work out the whole body, even if it's late in the night.

The thing is, when you understand how important exercise is to your health, and you decide to prioritize your well-being and how good it makes you feel, you will want to maintain that. If that entrenches itself in your mind, you'll never let it go. It's true that, at times, our partner, children, in-laws and parents or work become our priority, but you can only be there for them if you are there for yourself first. For instance, many Indian women tend not to take care of their health, avoiding having symptoms or signs of health problems medically investigated. '*Mujhe toh kuch nahi hone wala hai* [Nothing is going to happen to me]!' is often illogically said, as if one can just turn a blind eye and will these things away. It shouldn't be a surprise then, to be told of a diagnosis that family and friends say they're very shocked about. Years of neglect add up. Spiritually too, it is wrong to not take care of yourself. You are as much a spiritual being as your loved ones are. God has made you as much as he has made the rest of them. It's your dharma or spiritual duty to put yourself at least equal to everybody else, if not first.

What's in it for Me?

Your greatest reward from fitness is the outcome—when you see yourself looking leaner, weighing less or when you realize you have more energy, better muscle definition and cuts that you didn't have earlier, and are able to wear clothes that you couldn't fit into before, you become a convert. You *feel* really good. However, please do not go and reward yourself with a cookie, ice cream, cake, etc.—that would ruin everything you just worked so hard for. Always remember that the way you look and feel is because of your fitness routine and self-discipline. Nothing is ever going to taste as good as being fit feels!

4

Facial Fitness and Anti-Ageing Exercises

Facelift through exercise

Your face is your calling card! Your very identity. The sole reason I know you to be you, and you know me to be me. I've often wondered why most workouts are only restricted to parts of the body neck down. Does the face not deserve some attention too? The most important jewel in your crown no less! Incidentally, it is the first to bear the brunt of ageing, with the initial signs beginning to appear on the face as early as our twenties. Depending on genes and lifestyle, one may see deep wrinkles, fine lines, dark undereye circles, puffy eyes, crow's feet, laugh lines, jowls, a double chin, neck lines, furrows and droopy eyelids, all of which add years to our appearance.

Personally, I find it disturbing to see many people— even those just in their teens and twenties—getting all sorts of invasive surgeries, Botox, lifts and tucks done. Even if you ignore the fact that these are expensive, think of the risks and possible complications when undergoing anaesthesia for these procedures. Often enough, these can—and do—go very, very wrong. The *Deccan Herald* reported Indian actor Anushka Sharma's lip job that didn't go ideally, and that she was massively trolled for it. The same article reported on Rakhi Sawant that she is 'now better known for her ruined liposuction and implants'.[4] The *Hindustan Times* news item, 'Pop icon Madonna desperate to reverse plastic surgery' says it all.[5] CBS News reported about Michael Jackson, 'A whittled-down nose, lightened skin, an unnatural cleft in the chin, a chin implant, lip augmentation and God knows what else—Michael Jackson was a classic case of body dysmorphic disorder [BDD], Dr Youn says.'[6] The list of cosmetic surgeries gone drastically wrong goes on and on. What's equally worrisome is the notion of the damage these young lives are doing to themselves— mentally, psychologically and emotionally. I shudder to think what thoughts a young person's mind would be entertaining to the point that he/she is willing to go under the knife. How much must his/her self-esteem be suffering for a youngster to go through with this?

One of the best compliments I've ever received is when somebody I was just introduced to, gaped at me and said in utter amazement, 'You look like you have a 1000-watt light bulb under your skin. How do you look like this?'

I simply answered that I practise what I preach at Body Art. I lead from the front! I know that our Facial Fitness Anti-Ageing routine truly rocks! One of our clients, Varsha, felt her laugh lines were getting more prominent over time. This, despite doing everything right in terms of nutrition, sleep, lifestyle, the right products, etc. Within two weeks of doing our Facial Fitness exercises pertaining to laugh lines (the Upper Lip Tightener, the Head Tilted Back E-Smile, E-Smile Thumbs Up, Vertical Smile), she saw a marked improvement. She's now been doing the same exercises regularly for the last seven years, and despite her advancing age, we can see that her laugh lines have not only totally receded but remain firmly at bay.

The cardio benefits of exercise include increased circulation, which means clearer, better and glowing skin. If you're truly fit and healthy, it has a way of showing from the inside out.

Facial Fitness comprises of effective, fast-acting exercises. It is a fabulous, natural way to arrest and/ or reverse the signs of ageing, and create firmer, more radiant-looking skin. The results show in less than two weeks. Even though these exercises are generally meant for the whole face, many of them cater to specific problems. For instance, the Chin Lift is to remove a double chin and to sharpen the jaw line. The Eyebrow Lift is to eradicate furrows on the forehead. Each issue can be tackled with just one or a maximum of two exercises, done thrice a week on alternate days. It barely takes a couple of minutes.

Having said that, it is important to understand that these exercises are in no way a replacement for facial products you might be using or a maintenance routine you might be following. Please continue to do what you are doing in this direction anyway. There is no substitute for good nutrition and hydration (a couple of litres of water a day), sound sleep (quality and quantity), generally staying out of the sun during peak UV ray hours, using a good sunblock frequently, following a proper cleansing routine, using good, reputed face care products, exfoliating periodically and ensuring you get regular monthly facials—all of these are imperative for good skin health.

How Facial Exercises Work

Facial exercises work in various ways and offer multiple benefits. An interesting thing to know about facial muscles is how different they are from other muscles in our body, because they are directly attached to the skin. With facial workouts, the muscles contract and they take the skin along with them, thus toning and lifting the face. The gentle push and pull of the exercises on the skin increases blood circulation, letting ten times more oxygen, minerals, vitamins and nutrients reach the cells of the skin. This sloughs away old, dull, patchy and damaged cells, leading to a clearer, healthier complexion that can absorb moisture more easily. It also helps in the removal of toxins, thus preventing pimples, scars, blackheads and whiteheads (unless there is a hormonal issue). These exercises also stimulate collagen production, making the skin look younger. In just a few months, you would have taken off a whole decade from your face without any cosmetic surgery.

The best part is, it is never too early or too late to start a facial fitness regime—these exercises are preventive as well as corrective. They can help get rid of existing wrinkles, just as they would help prevent them from developing. Think of it as a non-surgical facelift programme that can turn back the clock to give you bright, clear, happy and healthy skin—naturally!

Let's get going!

> **Quick Pointers:** *Do's and Don'ts of Facial Exercises*

1. While you can perform these exercises anywhere and anytime, try to set a routine so that you don't end up skipping them inadvertently.
2. Follow these simple exercises every alternate day.
3. When releasing each exercise, do it slowly on a count of three. This sort of 'negative' work is very important. What's critical is not to release the exercise all at once, but to do it a little bit at a time. This negative work is superlatively fabulous, showing quick results.
4. Breathe normally throughout, ensuring you never hold your breath.
4. Make sure that your hands are clean before touching your face.

5. There is no need to warm up before or cool down after these exercises.

6. It is better to remove all make up before doing these exercises.

7. Remove all finger rings.

8. For exercises that have any part of your hands in your mouth, it is better to wear light, plastic, disposable gloves.

9. It is a good idea to combine facial exercises with overall body exercises to give your complexion a great hue and lift.

10. Go gentle. Never pull or tug hard on the skin, which may instead speed up the process of wrinkles.

11. Negative work is the discipline to not release an exercise all in one quick go, but to do it very gradually, to help you get better results.

12. While each exercise requires the detailed number of repetitions, it is important to listen to your body and do only as much as it permits. It is best to increase repetitions gradually.

The Eyebrow Press

Works on: Strengthening the muscles of the eyelids and reversing droop.

1. Place the forefingers just under the eyebrows, then push them back and then upwards. (Images 1 and 2)

2. Hold this position while progressively trying to shut the eyes for a count of three—first slightly,

then somewhat further and finally completely. Hold in this strained position for a further count of three.
3. Next, do the steps in reverse by slowly trying to open the eyes—first partly, then slightly more and finally entirely.
4. Repeat two to three times.

The Eyebrow Lift

Works on: Getting rid of furrows and lines on the forehead. Has a great Botox-like effect.

1. Lift the eyebrows upward and open the eyes wider and wider with each count. On count 1, open the eyes as if you are slightly surprised. On count 2, widen them in further surprise. On count 3, it should seem as though you're completely shocked. At this point, the eyebrows should be as close to the hairline as they possibly can be. Hold here for a count of three. (Image 3)
2. Slowly, do the steps in reverse order, i.e. from fully shocked to slightly surprised, until you finally shut your eyes. Relax to allow the tension to drain away. Repeat three to four times.

The Chin Lift

Works on: Keeping a double chin at bay and tightening the jaw line.

1. Tilt the head back and press the upper and lower lips together. (Image 4)
2. Stay in this position while curling the tongue up inside the mouth and pressing it against the upper palate.
3. Begin to smile on a count of three. On count 1, smile slightly; on count 2, smile furthermore; and on count 3, hold the largest possible smile. Remain here for a count of three.
4. Gently release the smile in three counts: somewhat slightly on count 1, further on count 2 and completely on count 3.
5. Repeat two to four times.

The Upper Lip Tightener

Works on: Keeping the lips from drooping with age and reverses laugh lines.

1. Place the entire length of the thumb inside the mouth, between the teeth of the upper jaw and the upper lip (Image 5). Since the thumbs are inside the mouth, it's a good idea to wear plastic gloves for reasons of hygiene, during this exercise.
2. Suck in and press the upper lip back into the teeth so that the thumbs feel squeezed.
3. Hold in this position for ten counts and then release.
4. Repeat three to four times.

Head Tilted Back E-Smile

Works on: Strengthening the lower half of the face including the jawline, jowls, ends of the mouth, laugh lines, and the neck in terms of getting rid of a double chin, and having great definition and form.

1. Purse the lips together, tilt the head back, and up. Start smiling an e-smile, wherein the corners of the mouth don't go up to the corners of the eyes. Instead, the smile is more horizontal. Do this progressively for three counts, starting with a small e-smile at the first count, then a slightly larger one at the second, and then the largest smile at the third count. Hold here for a count of three. (Image 6)
2. Reverse the e-smile gradually, releasing in three counts.
3. Repeat three to four times.

Tapping

Works on: Improving circulation for clear, healthy, glowing skin.

1. There are three positions in this exercise: above the eyebrow, under the eyes on the cheekbone, and along the jawline. Tapping should be done with the padded part of the forefingers. The tap must be crisp and fast, like it would be if you were tapping to check the temperature of a hot iron plate. Make

sure the pressure is bearable and not something that hurts. (Images 7–11)

2. For the first exercise, start tapping from close to the centre of the forehead, above the eyebrow, later moving outward in four stages in total, so that four different points per side are covered, till you reach the end of the brow.

3. For the second exercise, start tapping under the eye from close to the nose, moving further away till you get to the tail-end of the eyebrow. Make sure the taps are on the bony part and not in the eye socket.

4. For the third exercise, start at the chin and move further away along the jawline in four stages in total, till you reach closer to the end of the earlobe.

5. Do twenty taps per point.

Chin Slapping

Works on: Sharpening the jawline and increasing circulation to get rid of a double chin.

1. Using the back of your hands, lightly slap the underside of the chin. (Image 12)

2. Do this for fifteen to twenty seconds.

3. Repeat one or two times.

Neck Circling

Works on: Sharpening the jawline and increasing circulation to get rid of a double chin

1. Place the back of the right hand at the base of the neck and swipe it up all the way along the neck and off the chin. (Image 13)
2. Follow this with the other hand. Each hand goes in a circular motion, one arm after the next, alternating continuously.
3. Do this for fifteen to twenty seconds.

Little Pinches

Works on: Improving circulation

1. Gently pinch the face all over to stimulate the circulation. The pinches should be tiny, and while hard enough to feel stimulation, they should not be hurtful in the least. (Image 14)
2. Do this for fifteen to twenty seconds.
3. Repeat once or twice.

Rinsing the Face

Works on: Improving circulation

1. Just like you rinse your face, splashing water from the hairline to the chin, allow your fingers to run over your face (without water). Spread the fingers to touch as much of the face as possible. (Image 15)
2. Keep air-rinsing this way, stimulating the face for fifteen to twenty seconds.

Taps (not to be confused with Tapping)

Works on: Improving circulation

1. Using the pads of your fingers, one after the other in quick succession, tap them all over the face, including the forehead, eyes, cheeks, nose and mouth. (Image 16)
2. Do this for fifteen to twenty seconds in all.

E-Smile Thumbs Up

Works on: The lower part of the face—the laugh lines, jawline, jowls and neck, reversing a double chin and chiselling the jaw.

1. This is an advanced level exercise that requires gloves since the thumb is inside the mouth. (Image 17)
2. Start by inserting the thumb directly up on the sides of the teeth of the upper jaw. The rest of the fingers are outside the mouth. Start e-smiling out in counts of three, pressing the corners of the mouth downward. Hold for three counts.
3. Reverse the e-smile to a count of three.
4. Do this three to four times.

Vertical Smile

Works on: The mouth, nose and up to the centre of the face. It is for many muscle groups including the mouth, laugh lines, the nose, and forehead.

1. The exercise is intensive and you could feel a muscular quiver as when muscles work too hard. It means the load is heavy on the muscles—go easy.
2. Slowly snarl by starting out small, then broaden the snarl some more and then do a full snarl. Hold for a count of three. (Images 18 and 19)
3. Release gently in reverse order to a count of three.
4. Repeat three to four times.

Facial fitness is known to:

- Reduce the signs of ageing.
- Strengthen the facial muscles.
- Increase blood circulation to the facial muscles, making the face glow and keeping the skin clearer.
- Counteract the effects of strained facial expressions.
- Release any tension in the face and neck.
- Develop firm, taut facial skin.

5

Hair and Ageing

Decoding follicular anti-ageing

Your hair is your crown—you never take it off! So much of our sense of looking good, our pride and self-esteem comes from having great hair.

The first sighting of grey hair on your head is never a happy one. With a direct link to ageing, it is a reminder of the clock that just keeps ticking—in some cases, probably too fast. While there are many who ace the salt-and-pepper or the silver-hair look and it's certainly a natural process, often—particularly if it's premature—it could signal serious health issues and it is best to consult a medical practitioner to rule out any ailments like heart disease or vitamin B12 deficiency.

Research shows that the biggest contributors to greying and hair loss are genetics, stress, lack of nutrition and sleep deprivation (in terms of quality and quantity).

To most people, arresting hair-ageing may seem like an impossible, uphill task. However, in my experience, making Body Art's 'Seven Golden Rules for Hair Health' a habit can remarkably and largely prevent greying, thinning of hair and balding. Since prevention is always better and easier than cure, those following the rules as a remedy should know that the strategy will help in reversal, especially of premature greying, only to some degree. This I say, even though I've seen many of our patrons who have diligently followed the rules successfully, noticeably and naturally reverse greying.

Body Art's Seven Golden Rules for Hair Health

A Good Hair Diet

Food and nutrition have a huge impact on hair health. It is not only about eating good and healthy food, but also about not eating foods that are bad and unhealthy. The five-point rule is to eat more fruits and vegetables, include a good rotation of seasonal foods, stay away from wheat and starches, switch to healthier grains (quinoa, barnyard millet, bajra, jowar, nachni, etc.), and ditch the whites—no sugar, rice or flour. Add a healthy mix of protein, fruits, nuts and seeds to the diet—particularly eggs, beans, avocado, spinach, berries, cashew, almond, macadamia, pistachio, chia, flaxseed, sunflower seeds and fatty fish like salmon, mackerel and tuna. (*More on healthy substitutes in Chapter 7: Nutrition*)

Reduce Stress

Stress and hair health are forever interlinked. *Telogen effluvium*—where the hair thins, sheds, lies dormant and later falls out at the slightest touch or while washing and combing it is a stress-induced hair problem. Stress can also affect the stem cells that are responsible for regenerating hair pigment, thus causing the hair to grey prematurely. So, the best way to prevent hair loss and premature greying is to reduce stress and improve your lifestyle. Use different techniques to switch off the mind such as engaging in hobbies, reading a book, being out in nature, practising yoga or other forms of exercise, spending time with those you love, improving sleep habits, bettering one's nutrition and being more spiritually inclined, etc. *(Refer to Chapter 11 titled 'Coping With The Natural Effects Of Ageing', under the subtitle, 'Reducing Age Related Anxiety'.)*

Improve Sleep Habits

A good, restorative night's sleep is important because it helps the protein synthesis of the hair. It also aids in the release of enzymes and growth hormones that are necessary for overall hair health. That's why it's so important to work on getting quality and quantity sleep. Learn to switch the mind off and engage in happy thoughts—especially closer to sleep time. *(Refer to Chapter 13 titled 'Mental Ageing', under the subtitle, 'Sleep It Off'.)*

Improve Scalp Health

The root of hair problems lies in the skin that covers the head. The follicle and the scalp impact the quality of hair growth, and hence it is important to keep the scalp clean, nourished and stimulated.

Try and avoid products that contain sulphates, alcohol and fragrances to improve scalp health.

A good head massage helps greatly and so does brushing the hair twice or thrice a day—not so much for the hair but more so for the scalp.

As one gets older, one might even want to consider UV technology—a non-surgical approach to stimulate the scalp, thereby invigorating healthy hair growth.

Another great way of stimulating the scalp is to run open fingers into the hair, near the scalp. Grab your hair there as you fist your hands and tug away from the scalp gently. (Image 20) Release and repeat again in another part of the scalp. Continue doing this to gradually cover the whole scalp. Do this for about fifteen to twenty seconds in total. Running nails (but gently) along the scalp for about fifteen to twenty seconds is another great way to stimulate the scalp. (Image 21)

Keep Fit

Exercise, especially cardiovascular exercise, speeds up hair growth by increasing the blood flow to the scalp and by promoting the circulation of oxygen, nutrients and minerals around the scalp. Also, when we sweat from our scalp, it helps to unclog the hair follicles, allowing for new hair growth. That's why sweating it out is extremely important. Genetically, if you are not blessed with good hair, you will have to try harder via exercise and nutrition in order to see a difference. *(Refer to Chapter 7 titled 'Nutrition For Anti-Ageing'.)*

Maintain Good Hair

A regular maintenance routine is important for good hair health. Wash your hair every five days with a shampoo that feels good, cleanses the scalp and makes your hair look healthy and shiny, not dull or dry. Use a good conditioner that has the same effect. Trim your hair every month to avoid split ends and dry ends. Avoid heat on the head from direct sunlight, blow-drying the hair too much, using a straightener, rollers or other heat-based treatments. Protect the hair from harsh chemicals and use healthy hair dyes which don't dry the hair. Always wash the hair with water that is at room temperature or is cool, never with hot water as it tends to damage the follicles. Avoid hair extensions as they put a lot of weight on the hair and roots, thus damaging hair health.

Nawaz's Beauty Tool: Fingernails

Our fingertips and nails are amongst the best beauty resources we've got. Scritching, a process similar to scrubbing your scalp in the shower (except that you do it when your hair is dry and a bit more gently), is known to promote blood flow, lift dead skin cells and loosen excess oils from your scalp. It's a sort of dry washing of hair to break up and dislodge any dirt and dead skin from the scalp. You can even keep your hair healthy and nourished by using your fingertips to spread natural oils from the root of the hair to the ends.

Also, rubbing the fingernails of one hand against that of the other (called *Balayam* yoga) stimulates your brain through the nerve endings to send a signal to revive dead and damaged hair follicles. It helps in reducing hair problems like hair fall, dull hair, dandruff and premature greying.

Don't Oil the Scalp

This may sound counterintuitive, but I do feel strongly about not oiling the scalp and hair in the traditional way, which is usually commonly recommended. From personal experience, I find this to be detrimental to hair health. Oil is difficult to remove and hence requires washing with a lot more shampoo, and more times too. Also, you often end up pulling and tugging at the hair much more than usual in an attempt to remove all of the oil. This leads to still drier, brittle hair and hair loss. Oil also gathers pollutants and dust in the air, and heavy oils can weigh the hair down. Besides, I don't see any benefit of oiling in terms of improving the quality of hair or quantity of it, except that the scalp gets a good massage during the application of oil. Oiling and then washing vigorously can strip the scalp and hair of their natural oils, thereby worsening the condition. Hair quality and quantity is far more impacted by what you put into the body rather than an external application of oil. However, some dry oils and serums can have great results when used on clean, dry hair.

6

Callanetics

An iconic, sweat-free workout for a taut, fabulously sculpted, north-bound body

Ever wondered why sometimes you see two people—both the same height, same frame, same build and same weight—one looks great and is the proverbial head-turner, while the other doesn't even warrant a second look? Sadly, our idea of a great body is being slim, toned and weighing less; and yet, many people who are all of that, still look about as attractive as a beanpole. Being beautiful requires a certain appeal, a body that oozes oomph and charisma. Having a great body means being skinny in the right places, but stacked in the others!

Over time, I have come to trust Callanetics for a lean, chiselled body that has the right curves in the right places. The outcome is quick and highly evident. It may sound a bit like an exaggeration, but the results make you look like you have been under the surgeon's knife—except that you haven't! It works, even as all else fails.

After my second child was born, with exercise, the right diet and time, I did return to my pre-pregnancy weight and size soon enough, but I felt I'd lost some of the oomph in my curves. They were just flatter and broader, rather than rounder and hotter. Post-partum depression is hormonal, among other things, but you bet these sort of major downers very much contribute to it! A few Callanetics sessions quickly sorted all that out and there was a miraculous reversal, right before my very eyes! Soon I was back to looking like a million bucks and feeling totally on top of my game once again. It was such a lifesaver! I can't praise it highly enough.

For years now, I have witnessed several such success stories at Body Art. People losing twenty-five kilos in a year, those with knee problems, hip replacement surgeries and other health-related issues all finding benefits in ways they did not with any other form of exercise. For me, that ability to be able to help—even in the most difficult states of mind and body—is just priceless.

Why It Works?

Callanetics works because the exercises are all about very deep muscle work performed in small pulses and not total releases between one repetition and the next. This means that the muscles never really get a break— they are constantly taxed through the session and that's why the results are better. Most other fitness regimes only focus on the surface muscles, and hence aren't always as effective in lifting, sculpting, reshaping and anti-ageing.

Callanetics, on the other hand, employs a layered series of precise, powerful movements and muscles without putting pressure on your heart, neck, knees or back. It is gentle, slow and non-intimidating. Exercises are intensified only when you feel ready for it. These exercises are ideal for men and women of all ages and builds. Since there are no jolting or jarring moves, it's safe for pregnant women, people with disabilities and those with medical and rehab-related problems too.

Gravity does us limited favours. Over time, things tend to move southward, even for those of us who are extremely fit, toned and taut. Callanetics is the perfect antigravity workout. The cherry on top is that, very often, many of the exercises are done with body parts being in twisted formation. This brings in the 'Wow!' effect on those who have been proponents of Callanetics.

Callanetics really is magical. It teaches you to work at your own pace, listen to your body, and relax. There is no best time in the day to do Callanetics—do it whenever it fits into your schedule. A session of just seven to eight minutes is good enough to feel energized and most people begin to see a difference in only a couple of days. The weight loss is just incidental and the improved self-esteem is an added bonus. That empowering feeling of being in supreme control of your body is such an unparalleled blessing.

Continue with it as long as you want to see the same fantastic body and result. You can do Callanetics all through your life. It is gentle, easy and no matter what your age or health issues, you will find it hugely beneficial. Based on age, fitness levels and health issues, workouts may change and there probably will be variations, but the following exercises are immensely helpful in general.

POINTERS

In no time, Callanetics can:

- Tighten inner thighs and create firm, longer-looking legs.
- Reduce hips and re-sculpt the butt.
- Tone arms and firm up flabby underarms.
- Flatten the tummy, reduce waist size and erase saddlebags.
- Improve posture and flexibility, adding grace and confidence to movements.
- Increase lean body mass in proportion to body fat.

Compound Upper Body Work

The Cross (Two Positions)

Works on: All the upper body musculature, including the arms, chest, back, shoulders and neck muscles.

1. Sit or stand in a comfortable position.
2. Hold your right arm vertically in front of you. Then place the left arm horizontally in front of the right one, with the wrists meeting each other, forming a right angle (making a plus sign of sorts) (Images 22 and 23).
3. Begin with pushing the right arm forward and the left arm backward. Keep the moves small and controlled, releasing partially (only about 50 per cent) in between.
4. Exhale when you push and inhale when you release. If you find this uncomfortable (as you might feel you are hyperventilating), breathe normally. Just be careful not to hold your breath.
5. Ensure the arms are in a steady cross and elbows aren't jutting outward or upward, nor drooping. The chin should be lowered and shoulders relaxed so that you don't negatively strain the neck or the back. The harder you push, the harder you work. Try to target a moderate level of intensity.
6. Repeat twelve to fifteen times, take a break and do it again.

7. Repeat on the other side (left arm vertical, right arm horizontal).

Another exercise position would be to hold one arm vertically and the other horizontally, but behind the vertical arm. Switch arms thereafter.

Compound Lower Body Work

The Pelvic Scoop

Works on: The whole lower body, including the butt, calves, thighs and the shins.

1. Begin by kneeling down. If you have a knee problem, use a thicker mat for extra padding.
2. Start moving backwards as if you were sitting down on a chair, with your hips jutting out and shoulders forward. (Images 24–26)
3. When you're on the low end of sitting, fall short of your hips resting on the heels.
4. From this position, tuck the hips forward or under. Shoulders go backward on top of the hips, the whole spine forming the inverted letter 'C'.
5. Look at your tailbone in the front of the body. Hold it here for a moment or two. Wind yourself upward, a little bit at a time, powering through the butt by squeezing the hips. Slowly move higher, but not completely up; fall slightly short of that to maintain pressure on the working muscles.

6. Flip the hips back out, and repeat. Inhale as you go down, and exhale as you come up.
7. Beginners and those with knee problems can do this on the higher end (i.e., don't go all the way down).
8. Repeat five to seven times and do just one set.

Please note: These are intensive exercises and you will most likely feel sore the next day. Therefore, a cool down including some full body stretches is strongly recommended to prevent this.

The Pelvic Rotation

Works on: The pelvic region, the full lower body including the glutes (butt), abductor muscles (outer thighs), quadriceps (front of thighs), hamstrings (back of the thighs), lower legs including calves and shins.

1. Begin by kneeling down. In case you have a knee problem, use a thicker mat for extra padding.
2. Sit just one notch back and from that position rotate the hips starting from the right, going back, then left, scoop forward in a way that the hips are tucked under and the shoulders are back on top of the hips and form the inverted letter 'C' with the body. Hold for a moment or two, and then repeat. (Images 27–29)
3. Do five repetitions clockwise and then go anticlockwise.

4. A tougher version of this would be to do the same thing by going down lower till your hips are just short of resting on your heels. An even tougher version would be to strap on weights right above the knees, beginning with half a pound.
5. Breathing is normal in this exercise.

Abdominal and Compound Lower Body Work

Seated Leg Lift

Works on: The outer thigh muscles, gluteal muscles, all the abdominal muscles—waist and rectus abdominis muscle, transverse abdominis, internal and external obliques muscles, abductor muscles—one side of the body at a time.

1. Sit on a mat with both legs folded to one side, i.e., both feet turned to the right and both knees to the left.
2. Bring your left leg squarely out in front of you. That way, the weight-bearing axis falls on the outer hip of the right side where it's required and not on the opposite shoulder, where it's not required. Hold your left ankle with both hands to feel more stable and grounded when you are performing this exercise, and also to avoid leaning too far over to one side. (Image 30)
3. From this position, flex the working foot (right).

4. Using your core i.e. keeping the abdomen very tight throughout the exercise, lift your right leg up. If you lift it too high or straighten it out too much, you'll end up with a cramp. Keep it low and bent at first. Hold for ten seconds or so.

5. Pulse up and down for eight counts. Exhale up, inhale down. Do not let the upper body rock or sway while you are doing this.

6. Next, circle the knee clockwise for eight counts and anticlockwise for another eight counts. Keep the upper body stable.

7. Slowly extend the leg out to a count of three. Bend it back in to a count of three. Do this twice more. Release and relax.

8. Repeat all of the above on the other side/leg.

It is not uncommon in this exercise to feel a cramp.* To release the cramp, sit in a cross-legged position, reach forward, placing your arms as far out as possible onto the floor, and hold for twenty to thirty seconds. When the cramp releases, get back to the same exercise, only at a lesser intensity—meaning keep the leg lower and more bent than it previously was.

---

* If you take on too much too soon, you will cramp. This means you overtaxed the muscles—they were not ready for that kind of load and so have gone into spasm. Never try to ignore a cramp and run through it as it ends up getting worse. You will need to stop and stretch out the cramped muscle in order to get rid of the cramp.

The Modified Bow Position

Works on: The back muscles (particularly the ones in the mid and lower back), gluteals, hamstrings and the muscles in the back of the upper thighs along with the quadriceps.

1. Lie on your stomach with your knees apart and bent, feet together in the air. Keep the hands behind the back. (Images 31 and 32)
2. Lift your knees off the floor while tightening your butt. Pulse it up and down. Head and shoulders must be lifted up too. Inhale while going up, exhale while coming down.
3. Do this about ten to twelve times, take a break and repeat the set. Those with lower or mid back problems should keep their range of motion smaller, keeping the knees closer to the floor and the upper body less raised.

7

Nutrition for Anti-Ageing

The key to healthy longevity lies in our gut

Early on in life I understood a very important thing about nutrition and wellness. If you want to stay in great shape, it is something that you must understand as well. Fad diets don't work. They are a total waste of time and energy and don't let anyone convince you otherwise. Just think of it logically: if some fad diet did work, then why would there be another fad diet at all? The very fact that there is always a 'new diet' that is all the rage, means that the earlier one evidently didn't work as hoped for. The truth is that to look healthy, vibrant, have a great body and clear, glowing complexion, even at ninety, only a healthy, balanced eating plan, combined with a healthy lifestyle, will work. Both in the short and the long term.

My first tryst with healthy eating began when I was in college. Even as a young girl, I did not have the energy to get through the day. I sometimes felt dizzy, weak and could waft in and out of bouts of hazy vision. When I looked this up, I learnt it was an issue of nutritional deficiencies and could be easily corrected with the right type of food. As with most other college-going kids, my meal plan had centred around what was available just outside college—vada pav, sandwich (street food), makkai bhutta, etc. So I changed my eating plan and began to eat better, healthier foods, and in no time, all of those symptoms disappeared.

The importance of nutrition came into sharp focus again during my pregnancies when my obstetricians asked me to step up my protein, calcium and folic acid intake, and avoid things that were detrimental to my health. Post-pregnancy, I realized how important it was to eat right if I still wanted to look and feel as I did prior to pregnancy. Otherwise, growing sideways and ageing fast were all too easy.

You must understand that food is medicine. It is that magic pill that people keep looking for all their life but don't realize it is right there in their kitchen. It is so healing and transformative, nourishing not only the body and mind, but also the soul. That's why the onus of leading a healthy life and having a great body lies largely on our ability to understand nutrition and make the right, smart choices.

The Link Between Nutrition and Ageing

As one ages, the body's caloric requirement decreases, but unfortunately the appetite remains the same. The basal metabolic rate (BMR) also decreases, resulting in less caloric expenditure as opposed to what it was previously when one was younger and their BMR higher. These are some of the reasons as to why most people gain weight as they age. Besides, with age, as the stomach acids reduce, digestion gets hampered and the ability of the body to absorb nutrients is reduced considerably. Additionally, there is muscle loss, which manifests as multilevel problems relating to appearance, strength, integrity of joints and the entire musculoskeletal system. Externally, our skin tends to thin out with age, giving the appearance of ageing.

All of this is natural—it is how the human body ages. To turn back the clock and delay the process of ageing, you will need to work on cellular regeneration at the right pace and in the right way. To start looking younger and more youthful, you need to work on the basics. Here's how:

Eat What You Love and Love What You Eat

Don't get rid of foods you love, you'll only end up craving them even more. It's just how the mind works. For instance, as a Parsi, I can't imagine not eating Dhansak. And, like every Indian foodie, I love my chicken biryanis, dosas, bhelpuris, sev puris, pav bhajis, vada pavs and all the local foods I've grown up with in Mumbai. This is our comfort food—our emotions are deeply associated with those foods and so is our emotional and psychological wellbeing. So don't eliminate the dish. That's like throwing the baby out with the bath water. Instead, just replace the problematic ingredients with healthier ones.

Break Up with These . . .

As a first step, clear your pantry of all the whites—white rice, white flour, potatoes, pasta, bread. They age you, make you put on bulk and cause a multitude of health problems and diseases. Don't make excuses or say 'just one last time'. Trust me, there are great substitutes for each of these whites. For instance, instead of white rice, switch over to quinoa, barnyard millet (jhangora), cauliflower rice[*] or sprouts rice[†]. They are low (from negligible to virtually zero) in starch. In fact, quinoa is a complete protein—it has all nine essential amino acids that our bodies cannot make on their own. Barnyard millet is a local wild seed (not grain), mainly grown in the hilly areas of Uttaranchal and other areas in North India. Low in calories, rich in fibre, a great source of iron and when cooked, this gluten-free millet tastes similar to broken rice.

---

[*] Boiled cauliflower chopped super fine into rice-grain size.
[†] Boiled sprouts chopped into a rice-grain size.

Next up, quit wheat and wheat products. They lead to bloating and indigestion. Chapati and breads are best made with the flour of grains such as bajra, jowar and naachni (ragi). For pastas, switch to quinoa or millet ones. Almond flour and quinoa flour work fantastically in desserts in place of white flour.

Discard white sugar completely. I eat dessert after every single meal. I always have. Instead of white sugar, I've switched over to healthier but safe sugar substitutes, such as stevia. This is a plant extract known for centuries in South America for its sweetening qualities and medicinal purposes. It has zero calories and may help lower blood pressure and blood sugar levels. Do note that many people dislike the taste of stevia, but the secret lies in the brand. You might need to experiment with different brands in order to find the one that you like.

Our favourite potatoes need to go too but can be replaced with sweet potato. Another fabulous find is the turnip and red radish—they're both super healthy vegetables and when you cook them, they have a very potato-like consistency and taste. Use these for all your Indian *sabzi* preparations and dishes like dum aalu or for the bhaji with masala dosa.

As for oils, use canola oil, which has Omega 3 and 6—healthy fats which are good for the heart, eyes and brain, and for cutting other fats. Another excellent option would be grapeseed oil as it's a great antioxidant.

> You are what you eat. There's no escaping that truth. As they say, what you eat in private is going to show in public—so eat wisely!

Know Your Functional Food

One can't emphasize enough the importance of eating fruits and vegetables every day. They are a source of micronutrients that our body needs for a myriad of functions, to prevent diseases and ensure overall health and well-being. Each of the fourteen vitamins and sixteen minerals required by the human body are either not produced by our bodies or are produced in very small quantities. That's why we need to find them in food or from the environment— like Vitamin D from the sun. It's imperative to know that each vitamin and mineral has important functions and their deficiency can create severe health problems and diseases. For instance, deficiency of iron leads to anaemia, poor immune function and even difficulty in working and exercising due to low oxygen levels in the blood. Add to that, weakness and light-headedness, among other things.

Bring in the Superfoods

'Superfoods' refers to foods that offer particularly great nutritional benefits and minimum calories. Many have been in our Indian kitchens forever. We have so many valuable superfoods that are more than worthy of that title. Take for instance undervalued foods like drumsticks (moringa), amla (Indian gooseberry), ghee, turmeric, curry leaves, jowar, garlic, amaranth seeds (rajgira) and others like green tea, wheatgrass, eggs, avocado, dark green leafy vegetables (spinach and kale), broccoli, and nuts and seeds which are fibre- and nutrient-dense. Fish like salmon, tuna and mackerel are packed with healthy fats and nutrients, so do ensure you include these in your diet.

Pump Up Your Protein

Bulking up on protein isn't just for the gym rats who want to build muscles. A key part of healthy ageing is eating more protein as well. It is one of the three macronutrients that plays a crucial role in cellular growth, function, repair and boosting collagen. It also builds immunity and balances hormonal health. With age, the skin starts losing collagen, becomes thinner, loses elasticity and firmness, often causing lines and wrinkles. Increase your protein intake by including foods like soy milk, quinoa, lentils, chicken, eggs, tofu, fish, nuts and seeds.

Get Those Fluids In

The importance of water for good health and wellness can never be stressed enough. From replenishing electrolytes, maintaining optimal skin, delivering oxygen and vital nutrients to the cells, helping digest food and getting rid of unused waste via urine and regular bowel movement and more—this elixir of life has a very exhaustive to-do list. Considering our bodies comprise of approximately 75 per cent water, it is evident that consuming more will do a lot of good for the skin and the overall lustre of a person. Our cells retain or lose water based on a variety of factors. When cells lose water, a person withers and ages—inside and out. The youthfulness, glow and plumpness is lost.

More water also means fewer wrinkles, improved complexion, reduced puffiness, tighter skin that looks fresh, soft, smooth and glowing. As a main solvent in the body, it dissolves minerals, soluble vitamins and some of the nutrients as well. In fact, water relieves fatigue and helps you think more clearly. It also prevents headaches, cramps and sprains, and lubricates the joints. It aids in weight loss, reduces hunger, helps you to remain full for longer. Because hydrated cells function more optimally, they end up increasing the basal metabolism—this means that you burn more calories, even when at rest.

However, with age, the sense of thirst is often lost, so don't wait until you feel thirsty to drink water or other fluids. Typically, two litres of water a day is ideal. In some cases, a little more is recommended, while less water may be advised for those with medical conditions like kidney problems or diuretic and bladder-related issues. In such cases, it is best to follow medical advice.

The Alkaline Theory

Most of our bodies are acidic. An acidic environment leads to inflammation, can be cancer causing and is a breeding ground for other diseases. Alkaline water has a higher pH level (pH 8 or 9) than regular drinking water and is believed to neutralize the acid in the body. Normal drinking water generally has a neutral pH of 7. The more alkaline our body is, the better it is for our well-being. Adding lemon to water is a simple way of making water alkaline. It is best to have this first thing in the morning so as to put the body in an alkaline state. For those suffering from cancer, it is best to install multi-stage alkalinizing water filters that control the alkalinity of the water in varying stages. Ideally start drinking alkaline water at a low level and increase the alkalinity gradually.

Smart Planning for your Snacks

Hunger can strike at any time and in between meals— you know that at some point, you (and your family) are definitely going to be peckish. A smart way to handle it is to make healthy snacks in advance and keep them readily available, at home or at work, in a place where they are easily visible. Seeing them while passing by them in the home/office, has the mind register that these healthy items are available for you when you next get hungry. That way, you don't pine for all the wrong things. I keep a big bowl of fruits in the middle of the house for everyone to see and have. There are jars of nuts and seeds (unsalted and unfried) kept out there as well, for quick, healthy snacking, along with bottles of thinly sliced, dehydrated fruits and vegetables that give the feel of fried crisps, but they are not. Great snacks!

I also keep home-baked quinoa or almond flour cookies lying around in the central area of the house. You could add vanilla for that pleasant flavouring or put in black raisins, even nuts.

Bake your own bread with healthy grains. The added advantage is that you can slice it super-thin, thereby negating the bulk you'd have otherwise consumed. To bake your own bread, you don't need a fancy oven. A small, regular home oven will do just as well. All you need is a bread mould. You could use your healthy bread to make yourself a delicious, healthy street sandwich at home, by filling it with an assortment of veggies (like tomatoes, cucumber, beetroot, sweet potato and onions) and smeared chutney. Grill it for that perfect taste!

On similar lines, my favourite RTI (Ratan Tata Institute) mutton patties (my comfort food while growing up) now get made at home, with the outer covering made with turnip or even red radish (instead of potato). A still healthier variant is making the filling with soy instead of kheema and it is baked, not fried.

Another easy snack is an omelette or the Parsi akuri, with the thinnest Melba toast made at home from healthy, low-starch, low-calorie grains.

Make healthy salads (e.g. beetroot, papaya or tomato with basil and mozzarella) and keep these ready-to-eat in the fridge.

What is key is to keep these things around the home as a habitual, regular thing and then healthy eating won't seem like an effort—it will become an extension of you.

> *That one extra helping at the end of the meal:* Remind yourself that, frankly, you don't need it. That little extra bit is not heaped on as a result of hunger, but out of greed, and it's that same little bit extra that's hanging around your body—in your inner thighs, around your hips, the belly, around your love handles, the back—which you so hate. So do yourself a favour and just don't have it. Instead, down a glass of water at that point. You'll feel satiated. You won't even want that extra helping anymore.

The Caffeine Alternative

As I write this, I am sipping on a refreshing cup of turmeric root tea. It's my third cuppa in the day: I have ginger tea in the morning, green tea post my workout (to keep the basal metabolic rate high) and cinnamon tea in the night. With this, I cannot stress enough on the importance of herbal teas and how they work to keep me looking and feeling great.

Unlike other teas, herbal teas are not made with tea leaves. Instead, they are infused with spices, herbs, flowers and other plant materials. The polyphenols in these teas load them up with antioxidants, which are great for fighting diseases, infections and inflammation. Enjoy them hot or cold, for either relaxation or to soothe your stomach, or even for their sleep-enhancing properties. Just make sure you create a lasting, healthy habit that will benefit your body and give you the boost you need to get through the day—minus the caffeine.

Fight the Demons

As we age, our immune system begins to weaken, and hence it's important to eat the right foods to keep the body's defences strong and running smoothly.

Include nuts like almonds, pecan or walnuts when snacking. These are packed with Vitamin E and healthy fats. They're brain food.

Add sunflower seeds, avocados and dark leafy greens too.

Citrus fruits like oranges, tangerines, lemons, limes and grapefruit are great to produce antibodies that fight infection.

Papaya, red and green peppers, kiwi, broccoli, strawberries and cantaloupe have a higher amount of Vitamin C.

Include eggs, as they provide Vitamin D, which when combined with Vitamin C, boosts the immune system to fight off colds and the flu.

Ground flaxseeds have a host of health benefits, including antioxidant properties. So, it's a good idea to add a tablespoon of it to your meal.

Garlic and onions are great, and so is ginger, which helps keep inflammation in check. Make a cup of freshly grated ginger tea or add ginger juliennes to your salad or smoothies.

Green tea is fabulous. It has flavonoids and amino acid L-theanine—known for anti-inflammatory effects.

Herbs and spices like black peppercorn, turmeric and cinnamon are great to fight off infections and inflammation.

Raw honey works as an anti-bacterial that kills germs while boosting the immune system.

Mushrooms, spinach and broccoli are also superfoods for the immune system.

Yoghurt and probiotics like pickles, traditional buttermilk, kefir, sauerkraut, kombucha and kimchi are crucial for the development of the immune system and must be taken regularly to balance the gut health— something that takes a beating with age as the levels of natural bacteria in the gut are reduced.

When we pack our diets with these foods that are loaded with antioxidants, healthy fats and essential nutrients, the skin is often the first to show positive results. Meanwhile, the rest of the body will thank you for it. These foods are rightly called anti-ageing foods.

Don't listen to a nutritionist who says:

Eat only three square meals a day. Do not make this mistake! This reminds me of the old adage:
'No hope of escape,
No chance for the cheater,
The squarer the meal,
The rounder the eater.'

Ideally you should be snacking on healthy foods in between meals. You won't put on extra weight that way. Sticking to only three square meals is going to make you round because when you know you're going to have a large gap between one meal and the next, it's only natural to tend to overeat! There's your extra body weight right there!

Stick with soup and salad. No one—not even the nutritionist who has recommended it to you—has gladly grown up on soup and salad! Don't try to skirt the comfort foods you've eaten all your life. They're of paramount importance mentally, emotionally and psychologically. You just can't separate physical health from your mental, emotional and psychological well-being. I love my Parsi Dhansak—I just switch out the problematic ingredients. Rice is switched for quinoa. Sprout rice or cauliflower rice are other great options for rice. The kebabs with the Dhansak are baked, not fried; the potatoes are switched with turnip, the skin of the meat is removed before cooking (as it contains a high level of fat). The dal in itself is very healthy because it's a mash of healthy pulses and many vegetables, as is the kachumbar. I skip the fried onions.

Anti-Ageing Foods

Ageing is the process that occurs when the body cells fall prey to external elements and wither. If the body's cells remain well-oxygenated and healthy, ageing can be postponed. Certain foods can help in preventing cell degeneration.

Top ten anti-ageing foods that help regain vigour and vitality, keep the weight low and fight disease:

1. **Avocado**: This is one of the most alkalizing foods available. Avocados are very high in Vitamin E, which is essential for glowing skin and shiny hair. It also helps in keeping wrinkles off your face.
2. **Berries**: All berries, especially gooseberries, are very rich in Vitamin C and therefore, are highly useful to the body. Vitamin C helps in proper blood circulation and provides minerals and salts to all the body parts. Needless to say, this helps the body fight against ageing and keep fit. Berries are great antioxidants. The blueberry is considered to be the 'king of the berries', as it has the maximum nutritional benefits.

3. **Green vegetables**: Broccoli, spinach, lettuce, salad leaves and other such greens are highly beneficial for the body. Not only do they help keep the body weight low, but also help fight toxins. Fighting toxins is important because a highly toxic body is like a magnet for all kinds of diseases that can and do harm the body.

4. **Garlic**: This is one of the most important foods provided to us by nature. The benefits of garlic are numerous. It helps prevent cell degeneration, assists in keeping the blood thin and also prevents heart disease. It is most beneficial when eaten raw.

5. **Ginger**: This root facilitates digestion, has many healing properties and is therefore essential for the body. Ginger helps keep bowel movement in top gear, thereby enabling good gut health.

6. **Nuts**: Almonds, cashew nuts, walnuts, peanuts, pecan nuts, pistachios, macadamia and pine nuts are like power houses of energy. Consuming nuts on a daily basis will fight that lethargic feeling and fill the body with immense energy. They are brain food. They fight diseases such as heart disease and cancer, and are rich in the omegas or good fats.

7. **Yoghurt**: Yoghurt is rich in important minerals like potassium, calcium, protein and the Vitamin B group. Apart from these, what makes yoghurt one of the most powerful foods is the presence of live bacteria in it. This bacteria helps the absorption of nutrients in the intestines and stabilizes the immune

system. Yoghurt consumption has been linked to a lowered body weight.

8. **Melons:** Watermelon and muskmelon not only have an alkalizing effect on the body, but also provide the body with the essential fluids that it needs to perform various tasks.

9. **Whole grain pasta and brown rice:** Starches are long-term energy foods and should never be given up unless you want to invite trouble. Substitute white and wheat pasta as well as rice with quinoa pasta and barnyard millet, and you will instantly feel the difference in your energy levels.

10. **Water:** Nothing compares to water. Stay away from those aerated drinks. Water is essential for our body. It flushes out all the built-up toxins. At least eight (ideally closer to ten) glasses of clean, pure, room temperature water must be consumed on a daily basis.

Vitamin / mineral	Required for	Find it in
Vitamin B7 (Biotin)	Extracting energy from macronutrients; it aids in cellular growth and repair, DNA repair, gene expression. Great for hair, skin, nails, and digestion.	Organ meats, eggs, fish, seeds, nuts, sweet potato, broccoli, avocado, spinach, oatmeal and bananas.

Vitamin / mineral	Required for	Find it in
Choline	Ideal brain and nervous system functioning. Regulates metabolism, activates pain responses, regulates the mood, maintains liver health, and reduces the risk of breast cancer. It is very important in foetal development.	Eggs, milk, meat, fish, poultry, broccoli, cauliflower, cabbage, beans, peanuts and sunflower seeds.
Folate	Cell division. DNA synthesis and repair. Neural tube formation and reducing the risk of cancer.	Dark leafy greens, vegetables, citrus fruits, legumes, liver, seafood, asparagus, beans, grains, nuts and seeds.
Vitamin B3 (Niacin)	Works in the body as a co-enzyme that has in excess of 400 enzymes which are dependent upon it for various reactions. Healthy skin, nails, DNA metabolism, cell communication, mobility, cognitive functioning and much more.	Fish, chicken, meat, brown rice, legumes, nuts and seeds.

Vitamin / mineral	Required for	Find it in
Vitamin B5 (Pantothenic Acid)	Aids cellular function, fatty acid synthesis and metabolism, hormonal and cholesterol production.	Fortified cereal, shiitake mushrooms, sunflower seeds, milk, potatoes, eggs, chicken and tuna.
Vitamin B2 (Riboflavin)	Assists many enzymes with various daily bodily functions. It is an important component in reducing oxidative stress and nerve inflammation. Animal studies have shown that brain and cardiac diseases, even certain cancers, can potentially develop as a result of a long-term deficiency of riboflavin.	Eggs, organ meats, lean meats, milk, fortified cereals and dark green leafy vegetables.
Vitamin B1 (Thiamine)	Crucial for basic cellular function and metabolism of nutrients. Promotes healthy hair, skin, heart and nervous system. Supports healthy digestion and proper muscle development.	Whole grains, black beans, green peas, yoghurt, fortified cereals, pork and fish.

Vitamin / mineral	Required for	Find it in
Vitamin B6 (Pyridoxine)	Helps in brain function, lowering the risk of dementia, Alzheimer's and cognitive decline. Turns macronutrients into energy. Forms new red blood cells and develops neurotransmitters, building the immune system and balancing hormonal changes.	Fortified cereals, chickpeas, salmon, tuna, dark green leafy vegetables and fruit.
Vitamin B12	Healthy nerves, red blood cell/ DNA formation. A key component in development and function of brain and nerve cells. Important in the conversion of carbohydrates, fats and proteins into energy.	Animal products such as meat, fish, poultry, eggs, milk products and fortified cereals.
Vitamin C	Collagen production. Acts as an antioxidant. Critical in keeping immunity high. Important for wound healing, bone and tooth development, and blood vessel health. Also helps protect skin from sun damage.	Citrus fruits like oranges, lemons, grapefruit, red/green capsicum, broccoli, strawberries, tomatoes, cabbage, cauliflower and potatoes.

Vitamin / mineral	Required for	Find it in
Vitamin A	Eye health. Builds immunity. Helps in tissue, skin and bone development. Aids in the reproductive process.	Liver, fish oils, egg yolks, sweet potato, spinach, carrots and dairy products.
Vitamin D	Bone and teeth health. Necessary for calcium absorption and phosphorus maintenance, brain health, mood support, the nervous system, muscle strength, and reducing inflammation.	Cheese, egg yolks, fortified milk, breakfast cereals, seeds, fatty fish such as salmon (with the skin), tuna and fish oils.
Vitamin E (Alpha-tocopherol)	Acts as an antioxidant. Helps in muscle growth, reduces risk of cataracts, and promotes healthy neurological function and immune health, amongst many other vital functions.	Nuts, seeds, vegetable oils, leafy greens, pumpkin, asparagus, mango and avocado.
Vitamin K	Blood-clotting, heart health, strong bones and healthy tissues.	Leafy greens, vegetable oil and soybeans.

Vitamin / mineral	Required for	Find it in
	MINERALS	
Calcium	Strong bones and teeth, a healthy heart; supports muscle function; helps maintain proper hormone secretion and nerve transmission.	Milk, yoghurt, cheese, fortified milk, tofu, sardines, sesame seeds, chia seeds, water chestnut and fortified cereals.
Chloride	Aids cellular health and maintains acid and base balance in the body.	Table salt, sea salt, seaweed, rye, tomatoes, lettuce, celery, olives and many other vegetables.
Chromium	Fat and carbohydrate metabolism and storage. Aids in proper brain function and enhances insulin sensitivity.	Broccoli, green beans and whole grain products.
Copper	Bone, tissue, brain, and heart health. Strengthens the immune system, forms red blood cells and improves iron absorption.	Oysters, shellfish, nuts, seeds, potatoes, organ meats, leafy greens and dried fruits.
Fluoride	Prevents tooth decay and important in bone structure.	Brewed black tea, raisins, potatoes and oatmeal.

Vitamin / mineral	Required for	Find it in
Iodine	Plays a key function in cellular metabolism as well as manufacturing thyroid hormones and maintaining thyroid function. It also assists other micronutrients in growth and development.	Seaweed, seafood, dairy, iodized salt and eggs.
Iron	Red blood cell and energy production, metabolism and growth/development. Critical for oxygen carrying capacity in the blood.	Organ meat, lean meats, seafood, nuts, seeds, white beans, dark chocolate, lentils, spinach, tofu and fortified grains.
Magnesium	Energy production; muscle, heart, and nerve function; blood glucose control; blood pressure regulation, bone health and blood pressure management. Aids in digestion. It's also often used to help with relaxation and/ or sleep.	Green leafy vegetables, legumes, nuts, seeds, whole grains, bananas, raisins and salmon.
Manganese	Plays a role in metabolism, bone and tissue development, free radical protection and the sex hormone.	Spinach, oatmeal, nuts, shellfish (clams, oysters, mussels) black pepper and black tea.

Vitamin / mineral	Required for	Find it in
Phosphorus	Bone and tooth development, metabolism, cell and tissue repair, and production of energy.	Beans, nuts, milk, asparagus, tomatoes, cauliflower, salmon, poultry and meat.
Potassium	Optimum health of cells, maintaining blood pressure; electrical conduction in the body; muscle, heart, brain/nerve functioning and digestion.	Apricots, raisins, potatoes, oranges, bananas, milk and spinach.
Selenium	It has antioxidative properties and maintains thyroid health, DNA synthesis, bone health, and reproduction health.	Seafood, Brazil nuts, organ meats, poultry and fortified cereals.
Sodium	Balancing body fluids and ensuring proper nerve and muscle functioning, regulating blood pressure and transporting glucose into cells.	Table salt, sea salt, pink Himalayan salt and black salt.

Vitamin / mineral	Required for	Find it in
Zinc	Supporting the immune system, production of proteins and DNA, healing wounds and optimum functioning in the tasting and smelling departments.	Oysters, crab, lobster, red meat, poultry beans, chickpeas and fortified cereals.

Macronutrients: fats, proteins and carbohydrates

The Quick Switch Box

Replace This	With These
Rice	Quinoa, barnyard millet (jhangora), cauliflower rice, sprouts rice
Potato	Sweet potato, red turnip
Wheat breads (roti, naan, breads, etc.)	Breads and roti made with flours such as ragi, jowar, bajra, barnyard millet, cassava flour, etc.
Regular pasta	Quinoa or any millet pasta
All-purpose flour (for desserts)	Almond flour or quinoa flour
White sugar	Stevia or a natural fruit sweetener such as prunes, dates or black raisins
Regular oil	Sesame, canola or grapeseed oil

8

Factors That Affect Ageing

Live your best life as you age

With every passing minute of every single life, we are all growing older. Even a newborn infant is growing older. It's simply inevitable. There isn't anything you can do about it. What *is* in your hands, though, is dealing with the changes with grace, living a happy, beautiful life to the fullest, staying healthy and feeling your best—at any age. Ageing gracefully is more about being healthy and happy than just keeping the wrinkles at bay. Start with the little things: sleep well, eat right, drink enough water, pump up the collagen, exercise, fix your lifestyle and stay happy. Let's call them the six golden rules of ageing beautifully.

1. Sleep Well: Happy Siestas That Heal

A good night's sleep is highly recommended for physical, mental and skin health. It is known to lower the risk of obesity, heart disease and stroke. It reduces inflammation, stress and depression, and improves focus and concentration. When we sleep, our body enters a regeneration mode, restoring the cells and tissues of our organs and systems. That's also why, when you are unwell, doctors recommend rest and sleep. In fact, many medications do have a component to help you doze off to allow the internal systems to regenerate and speed up the healing process.

Often, the debate is about how much sleep is required. This varies from person to person and can range anywhere between seven to ten hours. Those who say they can manage with two to three hours of sleep and stay fit are the ones who can drop dead of cardiac arrest or stroke, etc. They just keep going, going, going and pushing the engine, till it eventually gives way.

When you talk of sleep, both quality and quantity are important. For a good night's sleep, it is important to try to sleep at about the same time each night (syncing into the circadian rhythm cycle). It also helps to create a bedtime routine such as turning down the lights, showering, changing into pyjamas and brushing your teeth. Try and wind down in the evening and not do things that get you upset or excited. The process of winding down is different for different people. For me, these days, it is painting, composing little tunes on my piano, playing with and teaching my kids, writing articles for various publications, reading, watching a TV or Netflix show that I like. It is important to put yourself in the right mental, emotional and psychological state.

Staying away from screen time (mobile, laptop, iPad, etc.) at least a half hour before bedtime is really helpful. Some people find that certain soothing drinks help them sleep better (for example, milk with turmeric, chamomile tea, etc.). What's most imperative is that you switch the mind off from the day's problems, just like you switch off the lights at night. If not, you're just causing a situation where you'll be inept at dealing with the problems of the next day. You'll be five steps behind because you're groggy, you probably have a headache, you feel sluggish, you have brain fog, things are hurting and you feel constipated. So it's in your best interest to switch the mind off, don't overthink things and reserve the next day's problems for the next day.

2. Eat Right: Mind Your Diet

Healthy foods are the way to go when it comes to ageing gracefully. While we have a whole chapter on nutrition for your ready reference, you must know that the rules to eating right are as simple as ABC. Avoid solid fats for cooking, Bring on the fruits, vegetables and whole grains, and Cut out processed foods, refined sugars and unhealthy fats. Also, it is best if you quit smoking and limit your alcohol intake—they pose unnecessary health risks.

3. Drink Enough Water: Stay Hydrated

There is a huge link between water and ageing. Drinking enough water helps improve energy levels.

It also boosts the brain function and helps you age gracefully. It has been proven to keep the skin healthier and to reduce the signs of ageing. Our bodies are made up of about 75 per cent water, so know that a plump, rosy and blossoming tight skin is indeed largely all thanks to water. You've seen how in a cold climate, when you drink less water and stay out in the cold, your skin automatically starts shrivelling, making you look old and frail. Inherently, you know you need moisture—actual water to hydrate internal systems as well as moisturizer for the skin.

Regular, room temperature water (not hot or cold) is best. How much water you should drink depends on your thirst, activity level, how often you urinate and move your bowels, how much you sweat and your gender.

The Detox Water Myth

'Detox water' is water infused with a fruit or vegetable or herb—for example, strawberry, lime, cucumber and mint, apple and cinnamon combinations. The claim is that it helps you lose weight, cleanses the digestive system, keeps you energetic, increases immunity, helps you feel positive and good about yourself. The truth of the matter is that the infusion (whatever it may be) is so minimal that it will not have any benefit. What would truly help is if you eat the fruits on their own. Not juiced (juicing reduces the nutritional value and increases the sugar level) but just the actual fruit. The water on its own—without additions—will do you good anyway, by helping you with digestion, losing weight and bodily functions, keeping you healthy, preventing diseases and keeping immunity and energy levels up. In other words, avoid the detox water. Stop kidding yourself and keep the regular water intake up. Eat healthy fruits, vegetables, spices, herbs, etc. in their own form.

4. Pump Up Your Collagen: Boosting the Levels

Collagen is the key to ageing well. It is a substance naturally created in the body, which gives the skin the strength and elasticity required to maintain a youthful look. With age, the collagen production in the body reduces, which is why you see skin sagging, hanging, and wrinkles appearing. I don't recommend dietary collagen at all, because if you have a healthy diet—a good rotation of fruits, vegetables, nuts, seeds, healthy protein with starch and whites replaced—you get ample collagen anyway. The problem is that, after a certain age, the body needs more.

While there is collagen in protein that can help to a certain degree, we need to maintain a careful balance, because an excess of this sort of protein can

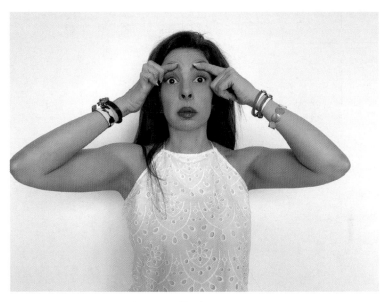

Image 1: Eyebrow press

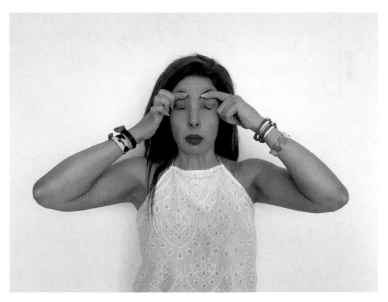

Image 2

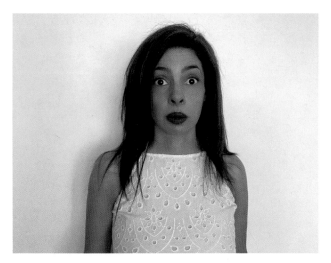

Image 3: Eyebrow lift

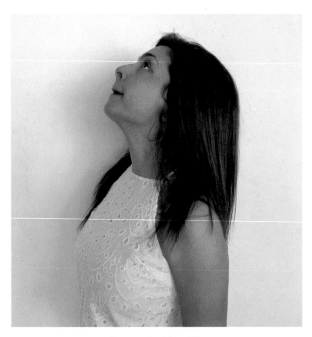

Image 4: Chin lift

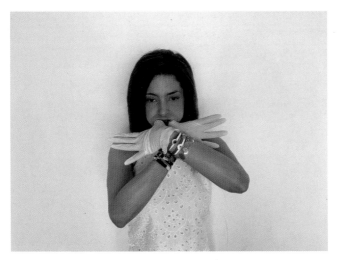

Image 5: Upper Lip Tightener

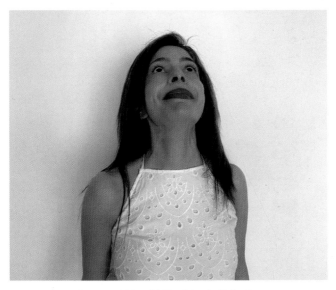

Image 6: Head Tilted Back E-Smile

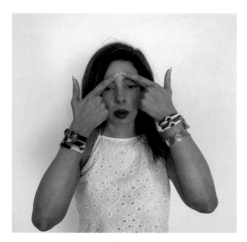

Image 7: Tapping

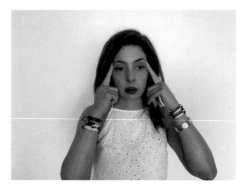

Image 8

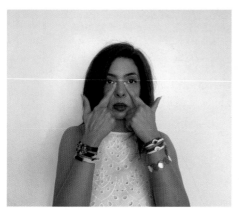

Image 9

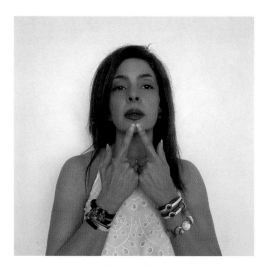

Image 10

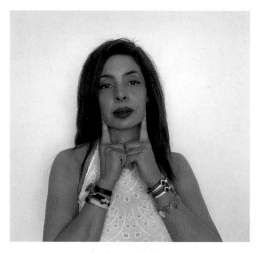

Image 11

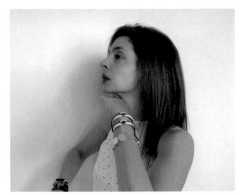

Image 12: Chin Slapping

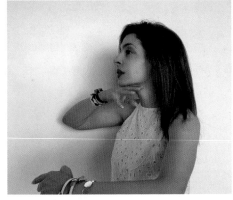

Image 13: Neck Circling

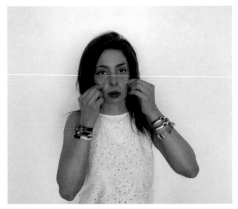

Image 14: Little Pinches

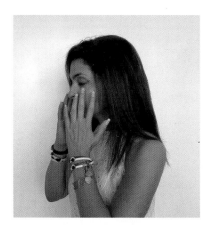

Image 15: Rinsing the Face

Image 16: Taps

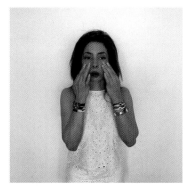

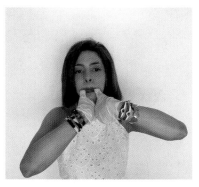

Image 17: E-Smile Thumbs Up

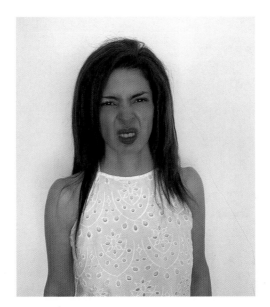

Image 18: Vertical Smile

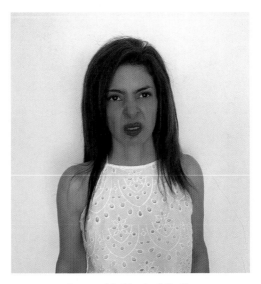

Image 19: Vertical Smile

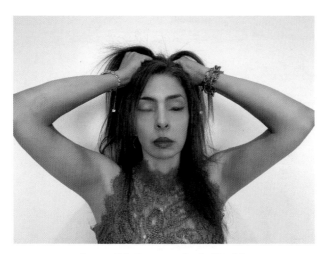

Image 20: Improve Scalp Health

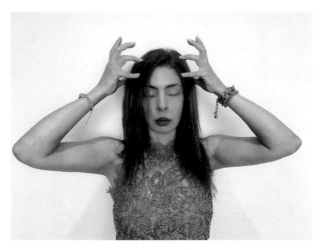

Image 21

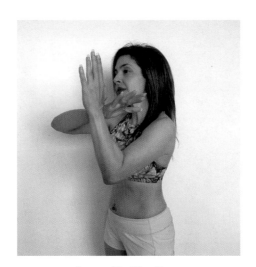

Image 22: The Cross

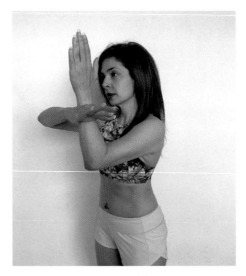

Image 23

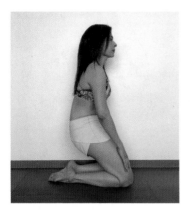

Image 24: The Pelvic Scoop

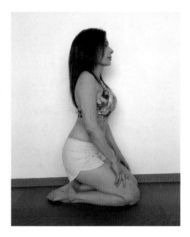

Image 25

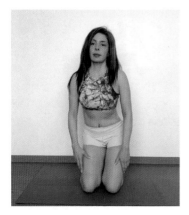

Image 26

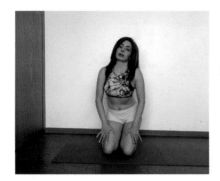

Image 27: The Pelvic Rotation

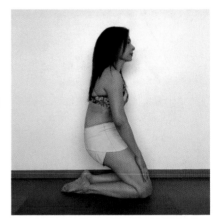

Image 28

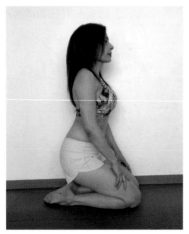

Image 29

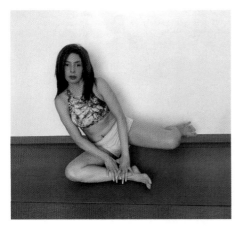

Image 30: Seated Leg Lift

Image 31: Modified Bow

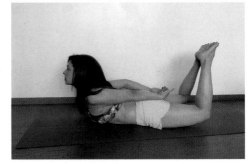

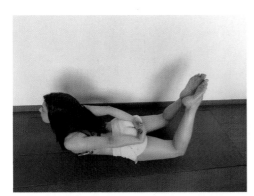

Image 32

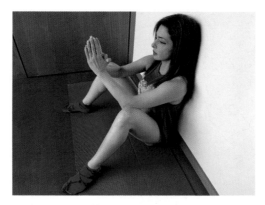

Image 33: Strengthening the Inner Thighs

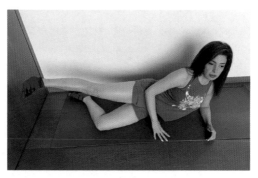

Image 34: Strengthening the Outer Thighs and Hips

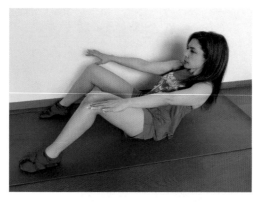

Image 35: For the Abdominals

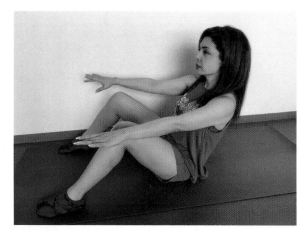

Image 36

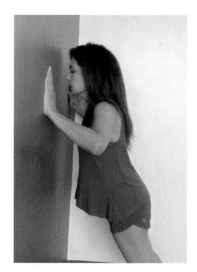

Image 37: Mini Wall Push-up

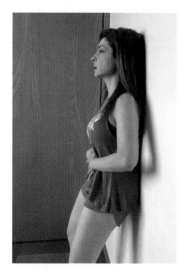

Image 38: Anterior Tilt Exercises

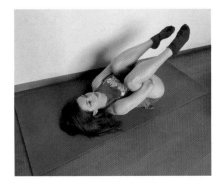

Image 39: Lower Back Stretch

Image 40: Upper Back Stretch

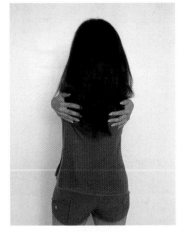

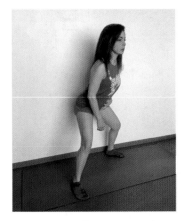

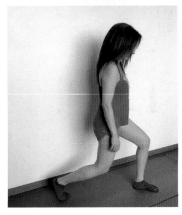

Image 41: Quadricep Strengtheners

Image 42

cause an overly acidic gut environment that leads to issues like heartburn, stomach ulcers and painful digestive problems. Also, the digestive system weakens as we get older and the stomach acids are not the same. Many elements including water, sleep, food and weakening muscles affect gut health. Collagen works at strengthening the connective tissue along the digestive tract. When damage is done to the barrier line of the intestine, it can cause a leaky gut—a medical issue where food and waste particles may be allowed to pass into the bloodstream causing inflammation, toxicity and leading to problems like gas, stomach cramps, IBS, etc.

A food item that is particularly rich in collagen is bone broth. Simmering the broth for a long time helps extract the flavour and nutrients of the marrow. Powdered gelatin is a cooked form of collagen. You could utilize it to thicken foods, soups, broths, etc. and it will quickly pump up the collagen quotient. Supplements are another way of doing this.

For the skin, there are various ways of stimulating collagen peripherally—facial exercises do it to a certain degree. There are also techniques that dermatologists suggest to activate the deeper layers of the skin, which naturally produces or makes the body produce collagen to get a youthful look. This isn't about going under the knife (I don't suggest that). I am talking of treatments such as different frequencies, UV lights, soft waves, etc., which stimulate the production of collagen. It's best to check with your dermatologist on the right techniques for you.

5. Exercise Well: Stay Physically Active

A sedentary life will only increase the risk of chronic illness. Regular exercise not only significantly lowers your risk of diseases but also helps you age with grace and retain your mobility longer. It lowers stress levels, improves sleep, skin and bone health, and lifts your mood. Depending on your health (best to check with your physician), it is recommended that you do at least five hours per week of moderate-intensity exercise or three hours per week of vigorous-intensity cardiovascular exercise or a combination of the two. Exercises can include walking, swimming, dancing and cycling. Muscle strengthening activities of moderate intensity using weights or resistance bands that involve all major muscle groups should be done for more than two days per week. Add to it a good measure of balance training at least once if not twice a week. In addition to this, whenever possible, go on long walks or hikes, take a vacation that involves a lot of movement and participate in a group exercise class.

6. Stay Happy: Mental Health Matters

The effects of stress on your body are vast, ranging from premature ageing and wrinkles to a higher risk of heart disease. Being positive and keeping your stress levels down, goes a long way in helping you live and age well. To keep your mood elevated, you can spend time with friends and loved ones, have meaningful relationships, a pet (if possible) and a strong social network. Reduce stress through meditation, breathing exercises and yoga. Practice mindfulness through meditation, yoga, tai chi and painting. If you're worried about something, talk to a friend or someone who will hear you out. If you find it difficult to deal with the changes that come with getting older, don't hesitate to speak to someone you trust about your concerns. Reach out for help to a family member or close friend. If that doesn't work, seek professional help.

Accept your age. Ageing is inevitable and learning to embrace it can make all the difference. Maintain a positive attitude about it—remember that growing older is a privilege denied to many. Do the things you enjoy. Fuel your happiness by taking time to engage in activities that give you pleasure. Spend time in nature, pursue a new hobby, volunteer—do whatever brings you joy.

The Way Forward

Ageing gracefully isn't about trying to look like a twenty-year-old—it's about having the physical and mental health to make the most of your life and enjoy it no matter what age you are. If you follow the dietary changes and exercises outlined in this chapter, drink a lot of water, focus on your sleep, pivot your thinking to positivity, you are setting yourself up to be the best version of yourself. The clues are there in the universe, everywhere you see—act accordingly. If your desire is to be healthy, fit, youthful and to look as good as possible, you will find that everything in the universe will lend its support. Like they say: if you have the will, you'll find a way; if you don't have a will, you will never find a way.

9

Pregnancy and Post-Partum Fitness

Making the most of a beautiful phase

So many women tell me that back in the day, when they didn't have children, they felt ready to take on the world. They were scared of nothing. But now, having had children, they are scared of everything! I can understand. When you're single, it's easy to be feisty, free-spirited, carefree and gutsy. When you become a mother, though, for some women, something inside changes—there is a constant feeling of anxiety about everything. It's true when they say that having a baby is like having your heart bouncing around outside of your body—it feels that precious and precarious, making you feel vulnerable like never before. And yet, it is the most beautiful feeling one can ever experience.

Several women are insecure about their looks and body after delivery. The truth is that women can look just as good and be as fit, if not fitter, after childbirth and we've seen some great examples of this time and time again. Put in the effort and the results will show. It's that simple.

To begin with, understand that during pregnancy, all the organs and systems of a woman's body are affected as they participate in a major athletic event—the preparation, formation and growth of a baby. The uterus alone enlarges ten to fifteen times within the span of thirty-six weeks and the rest of the organs shift themselves accordingly. So, after childbirth, when it is time to go back to square one, there is just one rule to live by: work out diligently and safely, improve your eating habits, increase rest, eliminate bad habits, and receive adequate pre/postnatal care—all of which will lead to a healthy, fit, beautiful, youthful you! And how do you motivate yourself to do all this during and after pregnancy? I'd say, by having self-respect, pride and not wanting to lose yourself to a decidedly downgraded version of your former self; by wanting back your looks, fitness, health and body shape in the process of having a baby, that should be more than enough.

Preparing for Childbirth

Exercise contributes towards improved endurance or stamina—a great asset during labour. It prepares you to use the correct muscles, apply the right amount of pressure and effectively relax those muscles which are not directly involved in the different stages of labour.

Exercise also increases your awareness of correct breathing and the impact it has on muscular efficiency. Mastering this ability to breathe with control is of great aid to a woman's management of her own labour. Besides, exercise helps you regain your original shape and size much faster post-pregnancy than if you didn't exercise at all during pregnancy.

Having said that, during the nine months, you really shouldn't be doing high impact activities, even if you have been on the fitter side. As the pregnancy advances, one's centre of gravity changes, one can get rather unsteady on the feet, and so one has to relearn how to sit, stand, walk and balance. With cardio moves, quick change-of-direction turns and twists, ups and downs and high-impact exercises that involve jumping, hopping, skipping or running, the chances of tripping, falling or losing a step are very high. Understand that you can't really see your feet and you aren't that agile or quick with your reflexes during pregnancy. Also, Relaxin, the hormone that is released by the body in preparation for childbirth to allow the ribcage to open with relative ease, is required in order to accommodate the pregnancy, to relax the ligaments in the pelvis and soften and widen the cervix. This hormone kind of makes you feel woozy in the head, slowing you and your reflexes down. With all the hyper-mobility that comes with the pregnancy-related flexibility, it is important to not push yourself too hard in your range of motion and stretches, lest you dislocate a joint or pull a muscle.

One Step at a Time

Keeping the trimester in mind, focus on the areas that could cause a problem. In most cases, physical work capacity decreases during the first trimester, increases during the second and reduces again in the third. As the production of the hormones—oestrogen and progesterone—increases, so does nausea, irritability, dramatic mood swings or that plain God-awful feeling. At the end of the first trimester, even when at rest, the heart has to work 40 per cent harder than usual (an extra 14,000 times a day), thereby increasing your blood pressure and body temperature. As the baby grows bigger and becomes heavier, the centre of gravity keeps changing constantly and the balance seems off, making it easy to feel awkward and clumsy.

After the fourth month, it is best to not lie on your back because of the weight of the foetus, which weighs down on the mother and circulation (and therefore the oxygen supply to the foetus is hampered or stopped). Sleep sideways or reclined or partially on the stomach but not on the back. With advancing pregnancy, the back also tends to arch, the neck gets stiff and calves can develop cramps. Lordosis or swayback, a common postural deviation during pregnancy, kicks in to compensate for a growing mid-section.

In all of this, the pelvic floor gets weak because of the growing weight of the baby and needs to be opened out to allow for a peaceful delivery. As a result, you may find the pressure on your bladder mounting and you might need to head to the restroom more often than before. (Mini pads for any slight leaking will help.) Also, with all the hormonal changes and the development of new vessels and ducts, breasts may become tender. As a result, the chest needs some help and work to avoid permanent sagging—it's important to wear bras that lend firm support.

How Much Is Too Much?

Pre- and post- natal fitness is different from normal fitness. Prenatal exercises are designed to meet the special needs of pregnancy according to individual case history and relevant trimester. Know that some of the internal systems (circulatory, cardiorespiratory, metabolic, etc.) are shared by the functions of pregnancy and exercising both. In general, the temperature of the foetus remains a degree hotter than that of the mother and the foetus relies entirely on the mother's body's ability to cool off. Because of this, you should be working out less than sub-maximally during pregnancy as your workouts build up your body's internal temperature. The core—where the foetus is—must not get overheated. Hence, it's best to keep exercises at low to moderate levels of intensity and never push beyond the prescribed limit.

Achievable Goals During Pregnancy

Cardiovascular fitness can be maintained and even improved upon during pregnancy. This will give you greater levels of energy to get through the day.

It is also important to increase muscular strength and posture during pregnancy, thereby automatically reducing the risk of injury and increasing stability. Strengthening the abdominals counteracts lordosis and helps in holding the pregnancy better. Working on our upper body strength can prevent bad posture and rounded, droopy shoulders. Flexibility is an attainable and desirable goal during pregnancy. Having said that, before you embark on any fitness regimen during the nine months, remember to fully understand the implications of pregnancy and the changes one undergoes physically, psychologically and emotionally, and the possible effects of exercise on the same. You should be aware of the common discomforts of pregnancy and the warning signs to stop exercising. Discuss them freely with your medical practitioner and trainer. Get information from your trainer about appropriate clothing and footwear. Take the trainer's inputs on the mode, duration, frequency, intensity and modifications of the workout, considering the pregnancy. Exercising in a supportive environment can reduce anxiety and stress while improving a woman's self-esteem and body image. Remember, healthy mothers produce healthy babies!

PRENATAL EXERCISES

Here are a few simple exercises you can begin with during pregnancy.

Strengthening the Inner Thighs

- Sit comfortably on the floor (or a bed if you prefer not to sit too low). Lean against a wall, with your legs apart, knees bent at about 90 degrees and feet on the floor/bed. (Image 33)
- With your palms together and fingers laced, place your elbows on the inner side of your thighs near the knee joints.
- While exhaling, try to press your knees together as you gently resist with your elbows. Release the pressure by about 50 per cent as you inhale.
- Start by doing two sets of eight reps each.

Strengthening the Outer Thighs and Hips

- Lie down on your side with the lower leg bent for back support and hips stacked one on top of the other. Lie on your lower arm. Lift the outer leg slowly as you breathe out and lower it with control (but without allowing it to touch the lower leg), as you breathe in. (Image 34)
- Begin by doing two sets of eight reps on each leg/side.

For the Abdominals

- Sitting with your knees apart and bent at 90 degrees, arms extended out and parallel to the floor, slowly

roll back halfway from sitting up and lying down while inhaling. (Images 35 and 36)
- Keep the chin close to your chest and your spine rounded.
- Slowly return to an upright position while exhaling.
- Start by doing this six to eight times and then gradually build it up to fifteen reps.

Kegel Exercises (to keep the pelvic floor firm and to counter urinary incontinence)

- Contract the pelvic muscles while exhaling and hold for a few moments. The muscles that you want to contract are the ones used during urinating.
- Relax the muscles while inhaling.
- Start by doing two sets of ten to twelve reps each.

Mini Wall Push-Up for the Arms, Chest, Upper Back and Shoulders

- Standing about two feet away from the wall, with your feet shoulder-width apart, place your hands on the wall at shoulder height and width. (Image 37)
- Bend your arms to the extent where the head is almost touching the wall. Don't let the back arch or your butt jut out, nor the pelvic region sag forward.
- Breathe out and push yourself slowly away from the wall without letting your elbows lock back.

Breathe in as you bend the arms and return to the start position.

- Begin with five repetitions and gradually build it up to fifteen.

Anterior Tilt Exercises (to counter lordosis, or swayback)

- Stand with your back against a wall, feet shoulder-width apart and about six to eight inches away from the wall. (Image 38)
- Press the mid-back into the wall and tilt your pelvic forward while doing this.
- Hold this position for a few seconds while breathing normally and then relax.
- Do this six to ten times.

Lower Back Stretch

- Lie down on your back and hug your knees into your chest. Hold this position for about thirty to forty seconds. (Image 39)

Upper Back Stretches

- Hug yourself really tight, rounding the shoulders inward and trying to walk the fingers as close to your spine as possible. Keep your chin close to your chest. (Image 40)

- Hold the stretch for twenty to forty seconds while breathing normally.

Quadricep Strengtheners

- Squats and lunges are a good way to strengthen your quadriceps. However, note that these should be shallow (in other words, done on the higher end), so as not to pressurize the knee joints which are already under much pressure due to the increased weight and demands of pregnancy. (Images 41 and 42)
- Start with two sets of ten to twelve reps depending on your individual strength and increase gradually.

POST-PARTUM FITNESS

Post-Partum fitness is even more important with regard to the long-term goal of ageing beautifully. Since most of it is really about losing the weight, fat and inches, you need to engage largely in cardio activities. Any full body exercise which gets the heart and the lungs working in tandem is what will do the trick. This could include aerobic activities like walking, dancing, aerobic classes, cycling, spinning, rope skipping, swimming, etc. Basically, mid-level intensity cardiovascular/aerobic activities of the sort (done in the presence of oxygen) as opposed to anaerobic activities (which are done in the absence of oxygen). What is important is that your heart rate increases, you breathe faster and more deeply.

Start by keeping it going at a moderate intensity for at least thirty-five to forty minutes (non-stop) and gradually build it up to an hour. Make sure you are well hydrated at all times.

One of the major concerns with regard to Post-Partum fitness is sagging breasts. It is therefore important to wear a full-support bra to prevent permanent sagging, which is anyway an issue due to the hormonal changes during and post pregnancy, weight gain and nursing. Another issue is that of leaking during Post-Partum. Often, the pelvic floor becomes weak after pregnancy. Because of the weight of the growing foetus in that area, the pressure on the bladder and kidneys is tremendous and it causes urinary incontinence (leakage). Therefore, the muscles need to be trained to function efficiently. Kegel exercises* are important to reverse the damage. Meanwhile, it is best to wear a panty-liner or a thin pad so that you feel more comfortable during exercise.

Most women are faced with the challenge of a loss in muscle tone and start feeling shapeless. You can do simple, full-body toning and total body conditioning exercises which will save time and get you to target

---

* Kegel exercises are great for strengthening the pelvic floor muscles. In pregnancy, these typically over-stretch and get flaccid, causing problems of urinary incontinence and other issues. Tighten the **pelvic floor** muscles, hold the contraction for three seconds, and then relax for three seconds. Doing two sets of ten each daily will show results in about a week to ten days.

the same goals, but in a shorter time frame. Every such achievement can be a big boost while you are anyway struggling with so many other things, like adjusting to mommy-hood, a new baby, sleep schedules, diaper duties, feeding, etc.

If you have Caesarean stitches, it may prevent you from getting back to exercising sooner, and it is best to start more gently, choosing easier abdominal exercises to begin with. Start with beginner level exercises while opting for simpler options, such as pelvic curls and pelvic lifts, rather than full crunches or sit-ups, as they're more challenging. Add them on at a slightly later stage.

If you are used to exercising, get back to it quickly and exercise as often as possible. However, if you haven't exercised previously or during the prenatal stages, start slowly, as the body is not used to it and won't be able to take on a sudden load. Having said that, know that eventually the goal should be to build it up to exercising five to seven times a week for ideal fat loss, inch loss, tightening, toning and regaining your figure.

Do Women Age Faster after Delivery?

Most women do. That's because they let themselves go—losing sleep by being up with their child all night, skipping on nutritious meals and not investing in themselves by exercising or taking care of their health and bodies. There may be additional stress from the pain of Caesarean stitches, too much interference from others or too little help; the new mother may be extremely tense and anxious at this point, which is very normal specially with first-time mothers. Stress does lead to ageing, as does lack of sleep. Reverse these triggers and things will improve greatly.

I feel having smaller goals is helpful. For example, in the second month after the new-born has arrived, families often host a naming ceremony, inviting family and friends. Tell yourself you want to impress these guests and have them say 'Oh! You've lost so much weight.' When you exercise, it will help with the post-partum blues*. Like I always say—do it for yourself entirely! You can go back to your pre-pregnancy exercises but start slow, easy, gentle and gradually take the intensity up. No matter how hard you try, it will take you about nine months to get back to where you were. Don't torture yourself for quicker results but don't give up midway either. You are the best judge of what is going on in your body. Keep adapting gradually to take yourself to the next level of improvement. That's how you get back to your normal routine.

---

* Post-partum blues is different from post-partum depression, for which professional help is recommended.

Drink a lot of water. Lemon water is good as it replaces the electrolytes lost through sweat, and which pregnancy and exercise both rely on. This is a simple method of replenishing electrolytes.

The happier, more positive, and more mentally active you remain through the pregnancy, the better off you and the baby will both be.

Do's and Don'ts

- Do consult your gynaecologist on recommendations and restrictions before embarking on an exercise programme.
- Preferably join a fitness centre and let the professionals tweak your workout for maximum result in the safest way possible.
- Always warm-up and cool-down for a minimum of five to seven minutes each to prevent injury. Include limbering and whole body moves along with stretches.
- Listen to your body and don't put up with pain and discomfort—they are signs to stop what you are doing. Remember that a change in the baby's position can also make an exercise comfortable at one point of time and uncomfortable at another.

- Breathe freely, deeply and regularly. Never hold your breath. Holding your breath can raise your blood pressure, cause headaches and dizziness and put too much pressure on the abdomen.

Prenatal and Post-Partum Nutrition

Pregnancy and motherhood demand an increase in the intake of proteins, folic acid, iron, calcium, Vitamin C, fibre and complex carbs for healthy foetal development and a fit mother.

Protein, the basic building block of every cell and of growth, can be consumed in the form of milk and milk products, soya, lentils and sprouts, eggs, fish, other seafood, poultry, eggs and meat.

A pregnant woman requires approximately 1200 mg (1600 mg for feeding mothers) of calcium daily and this can be consumed partly in the form of supplements* and partly in the form of food.

Since the iron requirement is high during pregnancy, a deficiency can lead to anaemia. Include iron-rich sources of food, such as watermelon, strawberries, black raisins, prunes, chicken liver, dark meat of chicken, spinach, dark green and leafy vegetables.

---

* Always consult your nutritionist/medical practitioner before embarking on any nutritional and fitness regimen.

Immunity can be low during pregnancy and post-partum, so keep it boosted with citrus fruits—Vitamin C in supplement form is recommended.

A common problem during pregnancy is constipation, so ensure you consume a lot of fibre in the form of fruits and vegetables. They'll also provide the nutrients and vitamins required to support the pregnancy.

Cut back on oils, sugars, pastries, whites, mayonnaise, butter and cream. Avoid anything which has an extended shelf-life—added oil, salt, preservatives, sugar and chemicals—they're all bad for health.

Instead of having three large meals a day, eat small snacks at regular intervals through the day. This will keep the weight under control and the blood sugar levels in check.

Drink water all through the day. Space it out well. Don't hesitate to drink water at night in the fear of having to wake up to go to the bathroom. Less water means reduced circulation, which can cause a cardiac arrest, stroke, etc., while sleeping.

10

Some Common Age-Related Ailments

Because age is but a number . . .

Friends and acquaintances tell me that the sight of a tiny person like me driving a large car, with my driver and bodyguard sitting comfortably in the back seat, makes for a hilarious sight. But for me, driving is the best functional exercise. It keeps you alert and your reflexes in top gear, working on hand-eye-leg coordination. It's a myth that functional fitness is only about fat and inch loss, flexibility, toning and mobility—it's got a lot to do with the brain as well.

Which brings me to the question: in your day-to-day functions, how fit are you? Are you able to sit on the floor and get back up gracefully at a moment's notice, without taking support from a wall or the floor? Are you able to get in and out of your bed without straining your back? Or does it always feel like you have slept badly, or that your neck is caught or hurting? Are you able to pick up and carry something reasonably heavy without complaining of having damaged your back and perhaps being unable to straighten up? Are you able to reach all parts of your back or your body with your hand? These are simple things but are very important tests of functional fitness.

As we age, functional fitness becomes increasingly important because, physiologically, the body undergoes several changes. There is loss of muscle mass and bone density, fat storage increases, the skin ages, the posture tends to get poor and often, health issues like arthritis, diabetes, cardiac concerns, cervical, lower back, hip and knee problems become common. Being functionally fit is the only way to deal with these age-related ailments.

Antidotes for Ailments

Cervical Problems

While a variety of issues can plague this area, exercises that maintain and help reverse certain neck-related problems include slowly turning the head from side to side in different ways. Keeping the associated muscles of the neck and those of the upper back and shoulders both stretched and relaxed while gently working on their strength when on an even keel, is critical. Ensure your pillow suits your neck and is not the cause of any neck stiffness, discomfort or injury.

Weak Back

People with lower back pain must first pay attention to their general posture, how they locomote and how they carry heavy objects to restrict injuries. In addition, doing low-impact exercises like bridges, knee-to-chest stretches and pelvic tilts can help in strengthening and relaxing the back.

Insulin-Dependent Diabetes

Exercise. There is no better solution than doing *at least* thirty minutes a day of moderate activity like brisk walking or biking for at least five days a week. Let this be your medicine and aim to arrive at a healthy weight by combining it with a nutritious diet. In no time, you will see a reduced need, or no need at all, for insulin.

Arthritis

Arthritis can cause severe pain, and exercise (strengthening, stretching and mobilizing) can hugely benefit the condition. Stretches and mobility related exercises can hugely relieve joint stiffness, especially during a flare-up. Walking, stretching, Pilates, water exercises, gentle cycling, strength training and flowing movements such as Tai Chi and yoga—which call for deep breathing and meditation—are extremely rewarding. Functional activities like pottery or gardening are also known to increase joint mobility and muscle strength.

Asthma

Asthma, emphysema and bronchitis can get worse with age. One way to improve one's condition is to go for gentle, low-intensity cardiovascular activities that don't overwork your lungs. To increase respiratory efficiency, try activities such as swimming, moderate-intensity walking and hiking, short-distance recreational cycling and gentle sports with short bursts of activity.

Weak Knees

As muscles and ligaments get weaker, it is best to age-proof your knees by improving your range of motion, enhancing muscle strength and keeping your weight under control. Avoid high-impact activities such as jogging, jumping and leaping and instead, go for low-impact ones like walking, cycling or step-ups. This should help in developing and maintaining the integrity of the knee joint. Do consult your doctor before beginning.

Hip Problems

It is not uncommon for senior citizens to face a variety of hip-related problems. Depending on the specific problem, severity and state of the individual, there is much that can be done via simple, quick-to-do exercises to maintain the integrity of the hip joint. The exercises strengthen the muscles while working on flexibility and mobility of the joint, among other things.

Coronary Heart Disease

Moderate and regular cardiovascular exercises as well as keeping a watch on your diet and lifestyle should help reduce high blood pressure, obesity, stress, high cholesterol levels and diabetes.

Urinary Incontinence

Besides lifestyle changes, pelvic floor exercises (like Kegel) are the best way to deal with this problem that can get worse with age.

Cancer

Exercise is known to lower the risk of protracting several types of cancer, including prostrate, breast, colon, endometrium, lung, amongst others. An added advantage of regular exercise is that it helps you stay at a healthy weight, because being overweight or obese is a contributing factor in approximately 15–20 per cent of cancer cases. Being overweight is linked to over thirteen different types of cancers.

Listen to Your Body

Remember that exercise and activity should be enjoyable and mostly pain-free. First, consult your doctor before starting on any exercise regimen. Next, ensure that you warm up and cool down with stretches before and after the main workout. If something feels wrong or you experience a sharp pain or unusual shortness of breath, stop. Switch to a more comfortable version or a more suitable exercise.

Other Ways to Increase Functional Fitness:

Eat Wisely

Nutrition-wise, as we age, our bodies need more protein for muscle-building and overall health. It's best to add about 180 gm of protein daily to your diet through a variety of lean foods like fish, chicken and eggs, and also beans and nuts. At the same time, make sure there are bright-coloured vegetables (think carrots, beetroot, spinach and broccoli) and fruits (berries, etc.) on your plate, along with whole grains (like quinoa, millets, amaranth and whole rye). Cut down on your salt and sugar intake for sure. *(Refer to Chapter 7 on nutrition for more details.)*

Live Well

As you grow older, take time to tap into your inner artist. Learn a new skill. Sign up for a painting class or learn to play the piano. Learn to play chess or bridge. Do the daily crossword. Have a positive outlook. Smile often and do things that make you happy and can brighten the day of those around you. No one likes grumpy oldies anyway!

11

Coping with the Natural Effects of Ageing

Dealing with the expected

What does ageing look like? Starting from the top, the hair begins to grey, there's thinning (for women; balding for men), dryness that makes it frizzy; it doesn't grow that much or that long either. On the face, ageing is all about lines—wrinkles, crow's feet, laugh lines, sunken cheeks, lines on the neck, a double chin, jowls. The skin thins out and elasticity reduces, making it loose. Since the largest organ in the body is the skin, ageing shows there first. But there are also other aspects of ageing—weight, cognitive decline, balance, bone density, appetite, bladder and bowel control and age-related anxiety—that aren't discussed enough. Let's try to talk about them at length here.

Skin-Tillating Woes

A full-body massage twice or thrice a week is hugely beneficial to counter the problems of ageing skin. Get it done by an experienced masseuse and remember that, aside from the technique, it is about getting the product into the skin. So, make sure the masseuse rubs the oils into the skin thoroughly.

Use one part of good quality coconut oil, one part aloe vera pulp (it's a cactus that can grow easily on your windowsill and has a lot of benefits) and one part of your favourite moisturizer. Before the massage, have a hot shower using a regular exfoliating scrub, as the heat of the shower will help absorb anything into the body more quickly. The exfoliation removes dead skin and stimulates the skin to absorb more moisture. Post the shower, wipe off water just from the crevices (don't wipe the body dry) and head straight for the massage. Since some parts of the body tend to dry more easily than the others (thighs, back, stomach, etc.) they will soak in the oil more easily; so, apply another round of oil there. Don't forget to get your hands and feet massaged too, as these are drier areas of the body and tend to show age sooner than other parts.

After a massage, don't shower—it won't feel sticky if the oils were massaged thoroughly into the skin. A shower will destroy the effort you've put in right before, drying out the skin again, alleviating the anti-ageing effect you just worked towards.

Apart from massages, here are other things you can do to keep the skin youthful.

- Remember that hydration has to come from inside out and so it is important to drink plenty of water.
- Keep the UV out and apply 100 per cent sunblock two to three times a day to protect the skin. Allow sun rays to fall on your skin only early in the morning or late evening.
- After a shower, I strongly recommend rubbing a cube or two of ice all over the face and neck. It has a great anti-ageing effect. Then apply good skincare products which you've tried and tested over a period of time. This is a very individual choice as products can be a hit and miss situation. For cleansers, toners, eye and face serums, anti-ageing creams, use upward and circular motions to rub in gently. Top it up with a 100 per cent sunblock and reapply every three to four hours during the day. Generally try to avoid touching your face till you're sure your hands are very clean.

Getting to the Bones

Osteopenia, another natural effect of ageing, is a precursor to osteoporosis (a silent killer). It happens when there is less calcium in the bones and you are at risk of osteoporosis but not quite there yet. Calcium is at its peak till the age of thirty to thirty-five, after which it begins to decline. The only way to compensate it is through supplements (women, continuously; men, from time to time in consultation with a doctor). Not all calcium ingested is absorbed into the body and hence, you need to get adequate amounts of Vitamin D, zinc and magnesium to help absorb the calcium and counter osteoporosis. Calcium-rich foods, milk and milk products, sesame and chia seeds and water chestnuts are some good sources of calcium. *(For more details, refer to Chapter 7 on Nutrition.)*

The Bulk of It

With age, our basic metabolic rate (BMR) slows down. While our appetite remains the same, our caloric output is not as it was when we were younger. It is far less. As a result, we gain weight steadily. Increased weight means increased risk of diseases like diabetes and health problems such as arthritis, knee troubles, back woes, compressed discs, sciatica and prolapsed (slipped) disc. This is because we first tend to put on weight in the mid-section of the body and that directly affects the back. A good example of this would be to think of putting on a weight belt of 3–4 kilos and to walk around with it all day long. It wouldn't take you too long to feel a strain. In this case, you can just take off this belt and relax. But when you actually put on those 2–3 kilos (or more) on the mid-section, you cannot put that weight down at all. No respite! It is going to have a debilitating effect on the back first.

With increased age, more problems will follow. *(Refer to chapter 6 on Callanetics for solutions.)*

All in the Mind

Cognitive health is all about the sight, hearing, thinking, learning, remembering and emoting. There are ample exercises I strongly recommend to keep yourself cognitively healthy.

For the eyes, make sure you move only your eyeballs and not your head. There's an old exercise wherein you begin by looking far out in the horizon and then look at the tip of the nose. Then look to your extreme right and look back again at the tip of your nose, then to your extreme left and again back to the tip of your nose. An extreme upward glance, back at the nose, a complete downward glance and back at the nose.

Another one is to circle the eyeballs clockwise, to the extreme periphery of your vision. Do this five times. Then reverse the movement (circle the eyeballs anticlockwise) five times. Then look as high as you can to the periphery of your vision and as low as you can, five times.

Other exercises include moving your eyeballs to look in vertical and then horizontal zigzags.

These exercises are great in keeping the eyes in good shape and order. By exercising the optic nerve, strengthening the associated eye muscles and improving blood circulation, eyesight improves.

For the eyes, ears and the mind, inversions are great. Plough pose, headstands and handstands are some examples. Even in hammock training—as taught in aerial arts, antigravity training, aerial yoga as well as the Pilates hub—the whole body is inverted, which increases the blood supply to the heart and does wonders for the eyesight, hearing, mind, hair and more.

Just like you exercise the body, it is important to do the same with the brain. For example, think of the telephone numbers or birthdays of twenty people you know, try to recollect twenty things you read in today's newspaper or do the crossword. Play chess! Play Scrabble™! There are so many ways you can effectively engage your mind.

Staying Positive

We've discussed how exercise improves mental health and makes you more positive and happier because we feel so much better about ourselves, our health and our energy. When you feel good about yourself, you are more likely to feel good about other things. You have the energy to pull people along, to lift their spirits and make things better in a very imperfect world. Yes, there'll be dark clouds, but the silver lining will seem so thick and shiny that the clouds will seem much smaller and easy to overcome. You will realize that every problem is a solution—very often an opportunity in disguise. That it makes you grow and improve, and takes you to a new level which you would never have gotten to without the challenge.

Exercise gives you all the tools you need to improve your mental health. Watch your thoughts and don't let negativity into your mind or negative people into your sphere. At the same time, don't depend on escapist outlets like alcohol or drugs to alleviate that little bit of a downer. These have long-term detrimental effects on mental and physical health. Stick to positive means of improving mental health. Do whatever you love, spend time out in nature, meditate, take time out to chat or meet up with friends, do whatever makes you feel good. Nutrition (Chapter 7) and sleep in 'Factors That Affect Ageing' (Chapter 8) too have a massive effect on mental health.

Sensory Impairments

For balance, proprioceptive fitness and functional fitness refer to 'Balance and Ageing' in Chapter 12.

Appetite-Related Malnutrition

An often-ignored age-related problem is loss of appetite. With age, there can be a change in the taste buds, dental problems, trouble chewing or swallowing, or blisters in the mouth. Consider appetite boosters and possibly supplements in conjunction with your doctor. If you find the big plate daunting, pack in the nutrients in smaller amounts and on smaller bowls with healthy food and drinks that include vitamins, minerals, protein and complex carbohydrates. Create a routine and eat with others (even if it is virtually on video chats) to make it a more pleasurable occasion.

Bladder and Bowel Control

One of the common problems that comes with age is bladder control. For this, working the pelvic floor with exercises like pelvic lifts, pelvic curls and doing the Kegel exercise (refer to page 94) ensures you don't have urinary incontinence. Do it every day and you'll see a massive difference. Follow the same instructions for bowel control by working on the muscles that control the anus. Do it about eight to ten times, two sets every day. Also, drink lots of fluid (unless there is a medical condition that restricts water intake). You can even improve your bladder health by cutting down on alcohol and caffeinated drinks like tea, coffee, chocolate and soda. Stop smoking and avoid foods that make you constipated. Eat foods which are high in fibre, like whole grains (the bran adds bulk to stool), fruit and vegetables. Avoid red meat, fried foods and fast foods, milk and milk products (don't worry, there are enough other sources of calcium), yoghurt being the exception—it's great for gut health, providing the right type of gut flora. Stay away from processed grains and their produce such as white bread and pasta, which are low in fibre and more constipating. Choose healthier grains such as bajra, nachni, jowar, quinoa and barnyard millet.

Don't hold your urine for too long, even if it means frequent trips to the bathroom and don't rush through it. Empty the bladder entirely and wipe properly from front to back as it avoids any infection getting into the urethra. Urinate right after sex as it helps to flush out any bacteria that might have entered the urethra during sex. For underpants, use only cotton or other breathable fabric and avoid tight pants as these can trap moisture in crevices and make bacteria grow. Overall, make sure you are physically active and exercise to maintain a healthy weight for good bladder health.

Reducing Age-Related Anxiety

Fitness is all about a good exercise routine, healthy lifestyle, wholesome nutrition, and your thoughts and emotions. It is holistic and you cannot separate one from the other. The healthier and fitter you are in all these arenas, the less anxious you will be. As for loneliness-related anxiety, work at having meaningful engagement with people in your life. Do whatever it is that you were born to do. It could be about giving back to society, engaging in whatever you feel strongly about, standing for a cause that you are passionate about or focusing on a hobby—something you couldn't do in your younger years because you didn't have the time. Just do it. It reduces anxiety and fears—contracting a disease, the uncertainty of life or everyday worries.

It's not that they are eliminated entirely but they are greatly reduced.

Steadying the Nerves

A simple exercise of squeezing a small ball (in the absence of one, even a rolled-up napkin will do) and holding that position for a few moments and releasing, is of great use in steadying the hands. Results are seen very quickly. Do this eight to twelve times every second day to begin with.

Maintaining Quick Reflexes

In the event of tripping, to prevent an actual fall and to catch our step in time, one has to rely on quick reflexes. I find a simple exercise that encourages hand-eye coordination and works on reflex action quickly, is to throw a ball against a wall and catch it each time. As you improve, throw the ball on different parts of the wall or even a bit away from you to challenge yourself further. Juggling a ball from one hand to the other is another option and very effective.

If you've lived well, invested right and saved for a rainy day, you realize that death is also a part of life. There is nobody who was born—animal, person, insect or plant—that does not die one day. If you have a healthy conscience, have done the right thing, earned good karma and are living in a state of well-being—

here and now—no matter how old you are and will possibly be, you come to a point where you feel you're good with whatever will happen going forward—your Maker will take care of you. Your faith will stand firm on this. And when you are in this good space, the fear of dying or of the unknown is lessened.

12

Balance and Ageing

Bettering your balance one step at a time

As mentioned earlier, with age, functional fitness becomes increasingly important because, physiologically, the body undergoes several changes. However, you need to continue to be physically adept so you don't suffer any problems while doing everyday tasks and that's what functional fitness is all about—your ability to do everything you need to do in your day, on your own, with relative ease and without any physical pain. Functional fitness enhances balance, endurance and flexibility and that's what will keep you going steadily in the long run. Incorporating functional fitness exercises in your regime trains the muscles to work together and prepares them for ease in performing regular, daily tasks. Since these exercises strengthen the muscles in the same way they need to work during a task, the risk of injury automatically reduces. The exercises can be done even at home with minimal or no equipment.

Do exercises such as regular squats, wall squats, frog squats, planks, plank variations, incline chest press, step-up and step-down, row, stationary lunge, single-leg lift, side plank, *Adho mukha svanasana* (downward-facing dog) and single-leg lifts. Make sure to warm up before you start any of these exercises. Once done, you can go about your day without straining or pulling any muscles.

Proprioceptor Fitness

As we all know, with age, injuries are common. It is therefore important to work on your proprioceptor fitness, which means being aware of the body and how it moves. *Feldenkrais*, which is the body's internal notion of movement and spatial awareness (of where it is in time and space), without having to necessarily look at yourself, is an important aspect of fitness. For instance, if you are doing a squat, you should know whether or not your thighs are parallel to the floor while doing it, you shouldn't need to look at yourself in a mirror. This kind of level of awareness is essential because it helps in working at the intensity level that is right for you and helps prevent injuries.

Another important aspect of proprioceptor fitness is balance. As you age, you tend to lose balance, often tripping, falling and not being quick with reflexes. You need to have quick reflexes for safe mobility. The mind needs to be trained so that, even when you lose your balance and are about to fall, you can catch your step in time.

To begin with, test your balance. See if you can stand on one leg and then move the other leg forward or to the side without touching the floor or tipping over. Doing this not only tests balance but is also a great way to develop balance. Another way of doing this is by closing your eyes and performing a simple task or exercise like a push-up or lunge or squat. You should be able to do it without having to open your eyes to see where the body is in time and space. It's an important skill to build. And just like balance and strength, proprioception is something that needs to be practised in order to see improvement.

There is a wide variety of exercises for the eyes, ears and mind that help with balance and awareness. Apart from these, other effective exercises include walking in the open, reacting to stimuli (obstacles and uneven roads) and change of centre of gravity calisthenics exercises. Bouncing a ball on the floor or on the wall (with or without a partner) can also improve hand-eye coordination. Practising inversions in hammock yoga, or a regular headstand, mat Pilates and also Tai Chi can provide an improved sense of balance and coordination. Surprisingly, certain video games with motion controllers can also help improve reflexes and peripheral vision—just make sure you don't get addicted to them!

Nutrition for Brain Health

Proper brain functioning is crucial for quicker reflexes. That's why you must eat a diet that nourishes the brain and the spinal cord. For instance, antioxidants (contain polyphenols) protect the brain from the negative age-related impacts of stress, which can contribute to cognitive decline. Foods like blueberries, raspberries and pomegranates are great. Add in Vitamin K-rich foods like kale, spinach, turnip and mustard greens, brussels sprouts, broccoli, cauliflower and cabbage. Soy foods, dairy, nuts and seeds are also a great source of tyrosine, which has a positive effect on our speed of reaction.

All in the Mind

Mindfulness exercises like breath work, meditation and yoga can play a huge role in making the mind stronger. They also end up improving focus, bring mental clarity and reduce anxiety. In fact, meditation is not about a quick reaction to any action. It actually helps in making you more aware of the entirety of a situation and you end up responding (and not reacting) with a certain level of overall clarity and awareness. That's why those who meditate will always have an edge over those who don't. Even if you do mindful breathing for one minute, wherein you close your eyes and feel the breath entering and exiting your body, it makes a world of a difference. Focus, pause and be in the moment. If your mind wanders (and it will), bring your attention back to your breath. It's simple and well worth trying.

13

Mental Ageing

Preserving and improving the grey matter as we age

As one ages, there tend to be subtle changes in the structure of the brain that affect the chemistry within and the functioning of the grey matter. This begins in middle age and as we head into our sixties, the actual brain size gets smaller, reducing the blood flow and the levels of neurotransmitters and hormones. The shrinking of the brain in its volume—particularly in the frontal cortex—affects memory, learning and other complex activities. As our vasculature ages and our blood pressure tends to rise, there is an increased risk of strokes and ischemia. Further, when the white matter of the brain develops lesions, the communication between the neurons is not as efficient as it once was, leading to the most common form of dementia, Alzheimer's.

Actually, by around the age of forty-five, the objective memory performance of an average individual lowers in comparison to what it was in their twenties. However, for most people, these mental slips are minimal and do not progress. For those who are affected though—especially if there is a family history—this is a major concern, because cognitive decline affects independent functioning. It can cause great anxiety and serious problems.

Becoming Cognitive Super-Agers

There is ample research and growing evidence of the fact that lifestyle choices impact cognitive health throughout our lives. Habits such as smoking, alcohol and drug abuse, lack of sleep, high blood pressure and high cholesterol are known factors that lead to cognitive decline. However, the good news is that these can be controlled and improved upon.

First off, exercise! In its impressive array of health benefits, the important one of staying physically fit is how it effectively helps deal with the factors associated with cognitive decline, including relieving insomnia, dealing with anxiety and depression and more. Remember the happy hormones we spoke about? (*Refer to Chapter 1, titled 'Exercise and Its Significance', under subtitle, 'Benefits of Regular Exercise'.*)

The next factor that helps is nutrition. A Mediterranean-style diet, which includes fruits such as avocado and blueberries, nuts, vegetables including the dark leafy ones, dark chocolate, whole grains, beans, seeds, moderate amounts of fatty fish, poultry, dairy products, and limits red meat, sugar, white flour and fried foods, promotes overall health— cardiovascular and otherwise. It lowers your risk of certain cancers and can protect against cognitive decline. Moderate consumption of alcohol (red wine, mostly) too is known to reduce the risk of cognitive decline.

Exercises for the Mind

As you age, performing mental activities gets even more crucial. In daily life, these can include reading, writing, solving math problems and crossword puzzles, playing chess and bridge, engaging in group discussions, listening to or playing classical music, amongst others. Try the memory game we spoke about previously, where you read the newspaper each day and later try to list twenty things you read. Recall the birthdays or phone numbers of twenty important people in your life. As long as you are stimulating the mind, one way or the other, it helps and does lower the risk of brain decline.

Keep it Social

Social interaction has a profound positive effect on health and longevity, especially with reference to friends, more than family. Research shows that people with strong, healthy ties to others are more likely to live longer, have better lives and are less likely to experience cognitive decline than those who are alone. So make sure to maintain a strong network of people with whom you can have meaningful conversations, where you support and care for each other and help reduce each other's stress levels. Call each other often, eat meals together, step out for a walk, travel if possible, catch up for a movie and generally motivate each other to live a happy, healthy life.

Sleep it Off

Next, sleep—in terms of quality and quantity—is important in ensuring overall health and preventing cognitive decline. The body relies on sleep, along with good nutrition and exercise, for a variety of essential, central functions that are controlled by the brain. While the right amount of sleep differs from person to person, experts recommend at least seven to eight hours of sound sleep a night.

Put Your Life in Order

Get organized—make notes, jot down what you need to do in terms of tasks, appointments and other events, and check them off as they get completed. Organize yourself in other ways as well. You should have a place for everything in your home—keys, glasses, medication, mobile, charger, bag, remote, etc.— and have everything in its place. Make this a habit, regardless of your age, because the better you manage and organize yourself, the better your memory is going to be. Training and organizing your brain this way regularly employs the grey matter, keeping the brain's functionality and efficiency sharper.

14

Spirituality and Ageing

Finding meaning to your life

When is a good age to turn 'religious' and 'spiritual'?, is a question I get asked often. First off, religion and spirituality, though confused with each other, aren't the same thing. Secondly, the truth is—regardless of what age and stage of life we are in, there are enough times when we wonder what our true purpose of being here on Planet Earth, in the life circumstances we are in at the time, actually is. It could be in our twenties, thirties or fifties—it doesn't matter.

I believe that all of us are just spiritual beings, currently having (taken) a human experience—and not the other way around. We have chosen to come here, of our free will, for certain reasons. In the quest to find the purpose of our birth and lives, some find it, some don't, some are perpetually lost. But the idea is to live life in the best possible way, being a beacon of light, positivity, hope, faith, love and goodness for ourselves, and for people and things around us. Our presence should be able to spark and spread joy, happiness and support, improving the things around us and being pillars and bricks for people and situations that need us or rely on us and can benefit by our help. In my opinion, there's no better way to work through and improve our karma.

Spirituality in Motion

The first step toward spirituality is being at one with Mother Nature. It is about appreciating the creator's creations, being mindful of ourselves and correcting ourselves along the way, because whatever we send out to the universe, know that it is coming back to us. The universe is a giant mirror—what we put out there, we reflect and so attract back. Hence, the idea is to become more truly available to this enormous energy field as we come closer to our maker. However, being more available doesn't mean detaching from the world, people, things, work, life, etc.—we are here for all of those things—but it is more about coming into our true nature. Slowing down, taking in the beauty of silence, knowing fully well that deep wisdom comes in silence—it whispers, it doesn't shout. It is soul-fulfilling, grounding, protective and purposeful.

Beyond Our Senses

There are so many parallel worlds and universes which we are aware of at different levels, but we often choose to just connect with Earth, through our limited five senses. However, I believe there is so much more. In fact, our senses can be deceptive. Think of the parable of 'The 10 Blind Men and an Elephant'. It tells the story of ten blind men standing around an elephant. As each person approaches and therefore assesses by touching the elephant from a different angle, each one concludes that the elephant is something different. The one who touches its sides calls the elephant a wall, the one who grabs a leg thinks it's a huge pillar, the one holding the elephant's trunk thinks it to be a snake, the one with the elephant's tail in his hand thinks it to be a rope, etc. The imperfection of our five senses! Therefore, the wise saying that you should believe only half of what you see and none of what you hear.

We should be more in tune with our other senses—our sixth, seventh and eighth senses. The sixth sense is our gut. The seventh is putting EQ together with IQ and trying to see what is really happening between the lines. The eighth is the ability to sense what's happening in our spiritual, parallel world that is reflecting here. When you marry all of these and try to synergize them in any situation, that is when you come closer to the truths of life—of matters of the here and now, and those pertaining to the beyond.

What Can Make You Feel Lesser Than

A spiritual leader once gave me the homework of thinking about what would make me feel 'lesser than'. For instance, would you feel lesser than if you had no education, if perhaps you couldn't speak English, if you didn't live in the home that you do, if you didn't have a spouse, if you didn't have a job, if you didn't have the assets that you do, if you didn't have friends . . . I found this to be a very deeply scathing and an eye-opening exercise in honesty, self-reflection and realization. We are born without any clothes on our back, and going through life we keep adding on a variety of things to feel better, more secure, more accomplished, and so on, about ourselves. Just like the very plain, unremarkable decorator crab—and the name says it all—that grabs every half-attractive thing it happens to find upon the ocean floor and attaches it to its shell to make itself more attractive. What happens when you put down the clutter? What are you left with? And how does that make you feel about yourself? Such a powerful exercise in self-esteem and so much more, I thought. That's just the start of the long journey into oneself.

Spiritual Resilience

In life, we have to develop many types of resilience, but the ultimate resilience really is your spiritual resilience, because in the many storms we all face in life, it is your lighthouse on a dark, stormy night and your anchor. If you have shallow roots, as the trials and tribulations of life progress, you are just going to be uprooted and washed away. When you stand for nothing, you will fall for anything.

Living is hard, not just for humans but for most living beings. You'll even see a tree fighting for its life—for sunlight, water—or suffering parasitic vines or fungus taking over, destroying and killing them in time. There is a fight in nature everywhere, even in what seems to be the most peaceful of settings. It's important spiritually to realize that we are all warriors. We have to get up and fight. Every rose comes with many thorns and if you are lucky to have a rose garden, guess what? It comes with that many more thorns multiplied! So one cannot bemoan one's challenges—spiritual, emotional, psychological, physical or whatever they may be—because it is what really makes us what we are. At times it is impossible to see and understand why we are being put through something, but when we look back, we usually find that what has really shaped us are the toughest of times. It's certainly true for me. I can now see that the worst of times *are* the best of times, because if they weren't there, I wouldn't have been where I am today. What breaks your heart will clear your vision. As Rumi said: The wound is the place where the light enters you.[7] They're master classes with the most valuable lessons for those wise enough to get them. The dichotomy of life.

15

Menopause

Focusing on yourself

Menopause, the natural biological process that marks the end of menstrual cycle, is often the most underrated phase of a woman's life. It is also the most ignored. One is said to have menopause when she has gone for a year without a period, and it can happen anytime in the forties or fifties, or in some cases, earlier or later. In the West, the average age of menopause is fifty-one years, while in India, it is forty-six years. Some women even go through menopause in their twenties and thirties. The age and pattern of when and how a woman reaches menopause could also be genetic. The other factors that influence menopause are largely to do with socio-economic reasons, marital status, stress and nutrition too.

Dealing with the Symptoms

Leading up to menopause—which could be over a period of months or years—one can experience hormonal changes which manifest in the form of irregular periods, weight gain, slowed metabolism, hot flushes, mood changes, depression, lowered energy, disturbed sleep, vaginal dryness, chills, night sweats, palpitations, thinning of hair, drying of hair and skin, joint pain, body aches and loss of breast fullness. However, these signs and symptoms are on a spectrum and can vary from woman to woman. Missing periods during perimenopause is pretty common and often, one may skip a month or two before it returns thereafter. Sometimes, the number of days that a period lasts are reduced too. Remember that one can still get pregnant during this phase.

It is best to meet the obstetrician or gynaecologist to find out more at this stage. They might prescribe important health screening tests like a mammography, a colonoscopy, bone density scan, check on triglycerides and other tests including a thyroid test, pelvic examination and eye exams too. These are great as preventive healthcare.

Natural bio-identical hormone therapy alternatives are a consideration during menopause, but it is best to consult your doctor before going for it. Honestly, menopause doesn't have to be a textbook case of difficult for all, because above everything, lifestyle changes can help greatly.

Treat Yourself Right

Exercise plays a big role in keeping the symptoms of menopause largely, if not completely, at bay. Daily exercise of about an hour per day—a combination of cardio and muscle training—is highly recommended.

Diet plays a huge role as well. Consume foods which are rich in calcium, because we lose a lot of calcium during menopause and get Vitamin D, because that's important in the absorption of calcium. Do a blood test to check if all the levels, including magnesium and zinc are up, otherwise calcium absorption is still a problem—it will get flushed out of the system.

Achieve and maintain a healthy weight. Eat lots of fruit and vegetables, drink a lot of water, and eat foods that are high in phytoestrogen. Consuming soy-based foods (soyabean, soya curd, tofu), seeds (sesame and flax), berries, oats, lentils, carrots, alfalfa, apples and beans is helpful at this stage. Avoid unhealthy foods such as the ones we have been speaking about throughout this book. The great thing about what is recommended in terms of diet and exercise, is that what is good, is good for everything. There are a million reasons why you should be exercising and eating right—there are no contradictions.

Love Thyself

Another important aspect that is often neglected at this stage is self-care. Many times, women make everyone else in their lives a priority and end up neglecting their own needs. Menopause is a time when, for once, they should focus on themselves. Know that it is okay to say no. Ask for help when you need it. Take time to apply that moisturizer after your shower, sit down to drink your morning coffee. Try meditating. Invest time in learning something new. Remember that self-care during menopause (also otherwise) is all about having a healthy, positive mindset, sleeping well, exercising right, looking after physical and mental health, and eating healthy so that you can give your body a chance to deal with the million changes while still rocking on and living your best life!

16

Accepting Your Age

And living life to the fullest

No living being has taken birth on Earth—in the human form, in the animal, plant or insect kingdom—that will not one day die. As a result, every single day that we continue to live, we inevitably come one day closer to the day that we will die. It is the ultimate truth and cannot be changed. Therefore, each day that we live, we are continually ageing. Time goes only one way and that is forward. That's how it is for all of us and has been, for all time. This is not something that we must 'begin' to fear in our thirties or forties. Ageing is a natural process and it starts from the day we were born. Even a new-born baby, from the moment it is born, is ageing.

What this book has aimed to do is to help you through the journey to live your life in the best possible way. Because even when you live in the best possible way, with optimum health, taking care of aspects like facial fitness, skin, water, nutrition, energy, sleep, lifestyle and other aspects that we have discussed in this book, the clock inevitably will still keep ticking forward.

However, you have a choice. Whether you want to move forward in life, ageing beautifully and gracefully, or let nature take its toll. Because it isn't just about how we look, but also largely about how we feel. It's a balance. It's an art. It's an ongoing process.

Dealing with the Ho-Hum

Don't get overwhelmed by all the hype about ageing. Once you start thinking about it, it might put you in a vicious circle of thoughts that can drive you insane. You can't keep thinking about 'what if' all the time. Instead, believe in the beauty of being healthy and happy every day—it will make your time on the planet so much more pleasant and enjoyable. Ageing changes everyone, so accept the inevitable. Don't let what you can't change get in the way of what you can change. The more you embrace getting older and wiser—you must appreciate its every tiny positive aspect—the happier and younger you will look and feel.

Write down positive affirmations to send gratitude to the universe and in return, you will achieve an abundance of what you want in life. Some examples of positive affirmations are: I am grateful for the life I'm living; I am grateful for my family and friends; I am grateful for my success; I am grateful for my strength.

Building a Happy Life

Get over the stereotypes about growing older. Let no one tell you what colours or clothes to wear or not, or if you should dye your hair, or get a certain treatment or not. For some reason, our society is very obsessed with pointing out the negative aspects of ageing or bringing someone down because they are in a certain age bracket. That's okay. There will be those who harbour prejudice against older people. Let them be. Tomorrow they will find that the tables have turned and they're now in the supposed 'older' person's shoes.

Build a circle of friends that are all about companionship, kindness and upliftment, and not about making you or anyone in the circle feel less than. Let it not be restricted to lunches and walks in the park—instead, find meaningful activities you can do together: things that you lacked the chance to do when you were younger. Make a list and start striking things off already!

In the end, no matter what you do, if you are happy at heart, it just has a way of showing—in the beautiful glow on your face from the inside out—and no one can take that away. From today on, every day that you wake up, aim for that glow. Let the sun shine!

17

About Body Art

Live while you're alive!

I was born and raised in Mumbai, and schooled at the Cathedral and John Connon School in Fort, following which I went to Junior College and completed my Bachelor of Arts at St. Xavier's College.

When I was in the last year of college, I was wondering, like most other kids were, as to what I wanted to do with the rest of my life. The obvious choice was law, since so many people in my family are lawyers. However, I veered more towards fitness, stemming from my own personal experiences when I was younger. Writing and psychology were also tempting options for me. Not having four bodies to accomplish all my dreams and wishes through, I decided to study law and get into fitness simultaneously.

I studied law at the Government Law College and graduated from K.C. Law College in Mumbai. Somehow juggling matters, I also went to USA for six months, where I got myself trained and certified in fitness via ACE (American Council on Exercise) and IDEA (International Dance Exercise Association). Having gotten some work experience, I came back to India. I then started up my baby—Body Art Fitness Centres.

I started small, in a single room, where I introduced the Aerobic Workshop group classes. Then I started basic routines such as step, high-low fusions and calisthenics. Over a period of time, I both pioneered and introduced many firsts into the country, such as choreographed slide training classes, choreographed mini trampoline classes, stress management classes, calisthenics, anti-ageing facial fitness classes and so on. More and more routines were subsequently introduced, such as Zumba, new body format, box-aerobics, cardio dance, sculpt, mat Pilates, partner workouts, Callanetics, muscle ballet, Swiss ball, NYC ballet basics, circuit training, chair workouts, functional fitness and others.

Thereafter, a traditional gym was introduced, followed by India's first full-fledged equipment-based Pilates and Gyrotonic Hub. Subsequent to that, aqua aerobics and aqua yoga were introduced, followed by spinning/indoor biking group classes.

The next introduction was of the aerial art studios where anti-gravity workouts, aerial yoga and TRX training is conducted.

While much focus has always been placed on individualization for every member, taking their health history, their fitness level, goals, age, likes and dislikes into account, personal training makes highly bespoke workouts that can sharply focus on the individual's goal.

One fitness centre grew to second location, a third, and so on.

In March 2020, when Covid lockdown struck us all and all our centres were shut, we went online and conducted our aerobic workshop group classes live online along with a large variety of personal training workouts such as kettlebell workouts, chair workouts, free-weight workouts, sculpt, power yoga, mat Pilates, band/dupatta workouts, ZUU animal walk workout, functional fitness, body weight training, book training, towel training, total body conditioning, ball training, yogalates, Gyrokinesis, yoga and *pranayama*, calisthenics, Callanetics, and more.

Members who over the years had migrated, moving countries too, had always lamented that they'd never found a place as good as *Body Art* again, no matter how many places they had tried out. They were delighted when we went online as now they could finally join us no matter where in the world they were.

Notes

1. The University of South Australia states that, 'Exercise is more effective than medicines to manage mental health'. Their researchers are asking for exercise to be a mainstay approach in managing depression, as newer research and studies show that physical activity is 1.5 times more effective than counselling or the leading medications; 'Exercise more effective than medicines to manage mental health', University of South Australia, 24 February 2023, https://www.unisa.edu.au/media-centre/Releases/2023/exercise-more-effective-than-medicines-to-manage-mental-health/;

The Harvard University states that, 'Exercise is an all-natural treatment to fight depression', and that 'for some people it works as well as anti-depressants'; 'Exercise is an all-natural treatment to fight depression', Harvard Health Publishing, 2 February 2021, https://www.health.harvard.

edu/mind-and-mood/exercise-is-an-all-natural-treatment-to-fight-depression;

Quoted from Medical News Today, 'Physical activity is 1.5 times more effective at reducing mild to moderate symptoms of depression, psychological stress, anxiety than medication or cognitive behaviour therapy, according to the study's lead author, Dr. Ben Singh.' 'Is exercise more effective than medication for depression and anxiety?', Medical News Today, 3 March 2023, https://www.medicalnewstoday.com/articles/is-exercise-more-effective-than-medication-for-depression-and-anxiety.

2. 'Strategies to Prevent Heart Disease', Mayo Clinic, 14 January 2022, https://www.mayoclinic.org/diseases-conditions/heart-disease/in-depth/heart-disease-prevention/art-20046502.

3. Goodreads.com, https://www.goodreads.com/quotes/978-whether-you-think-you-can-or-you-think-you-can-t--you-re, last accessed 3 July 2023.

4. 'Stars with cosmetic surgeries gone wrong', *Deccan Herald*, 10 April 2022, https://www.deccanherald.com/dh-galleries/photos/in-pics-stars-with-cosmetic-surgeries-gone-wrong-1098843.

5. 'Madonna's facelift fiasco: Pop icon to go Under the knife again to erase Grammy's face, insider reveals', *Hindustan Times*, 8 April 2023, https://www.hindustantimes.com/entertainment/others/madonnas-plastic-surgery-disaster-pop-icon-

desperate-to-reverse-botched-procedures-before-world-tour-sources-claim-101680962231027.html.

6. 'Celebrity Plastic Surgery Disasters?', CBS News, 4 January 2011, https://www.cbsnews.com/pictures/celebrity-plastic-surgery-disasters/.

7. Goodreads.com,   https://www.goodreads.com/quotes/103315-the-wound-is-the-place-where-the-light-enters-you, last accessed 3 July 2023.